Women 7... S...RAMENTO PUBLIC ...ARY
on Thund...
Cheese Fries, an...
Good ... at Any Size

tales
from the
scale

Erin J. Shea

Polka Dot Press
Avon, Massachusetts

Published by
Polka Dot Press, an imprint of
Adams Media, an F+W Publications Company
57 Littlefield Street, Avon, MA 02322. U.S.A.
www.adamsmedia.com

ISBN: 1-59337-328-7

Printed in the United States of America.

J I H G F E D C B A

Library of Congress Cataloging-in-Publication Data
Shea, Erin J.
Tales from the scale / Erin J. Shea.
p.   cm.
ISBN 1-59337-328-7
1. Overweight women—Anecdotes. 2. Overweight women—Humor.
3. Obesity in women—Psychological aspects. I. Title.
RC552.O25S445   2005
362.196'398'00922—dc22   2004022196

This publication is designed to provide accurate and authoritative information with
regard to the subject matter covered. It is sold with the understanding that the
publisher is not engaged in rendering legal, accounting, or other professional advice.
If legal advice or other expert assistance is required, the services of a competent
professional person should be sought.
        —From a *Declaration of Principles* jointly adopted by a Committee of the
American Bar Association and a Committee of Publishers and Associations

Many of the designations used by manufacturers and sellers to distinguish their
products are claimed as trademarks. Where those designations appear in this
book and Adams Media was aware of a trademark claim, the designations have
been printed with initial capital letters.

This book is available at quantity discounts for bulk purchases.
For information, call 1-800-872-5627.

This book is for all the Fat Girls everywhere and is dedicated in the memory of my mother, Catherine Hazel Shea, who claimed to have lost weight one summer by eating only Oreo cookies and playing tennis.

For the record, she told me that this was not the smartest way to go about a diet and I'm certain if she were still alive today she would tell you likewise.

Wish you could have seen this, Mom. I miss you.

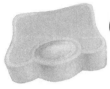

Acknowledgments

FIRST THINGS FIRST.

I can't believe I'm writing an acknowledgments page, because it means I've published a book requiring me to do so. Even if this book tanks, and you all rush over to Amazon.com to give it scathing, snarky reviews, it still happened. I can barely contain myself but will try my best.

None of this would be possible were it not for three people. The first is Amy Harmon, technology reporter for the *New York Times*. Had Amy not decided to write an article in August 2003 about weight-loss blogs and had she not interviewed me for it, I'd still be cranking this stuff out for free at my Web site. I like getting paid. Thanks, Amy. The second is my agent, Stephanie Lee, who two days after the *Times* article ran e-mailed me to ask what she now knows was perceived by me as purely a rhetorical question: "Have you ever considered writing a book?" Stephanie championed this project from its inception and held my hand through the entire process. She is as kind and funny as she is talented and wicked smart. The last is my editor, Danielle Chiotti, who put up with my incessant rambling, made this book sing, and didn't drop the project altogether when she made a title suggestion to me and I answered her by saying that I would rather repeatedly jam hot pokers into my eyes than use that title. A saint you are, Danielle. Thank you for being my friend and for dragging my ass out on a school night to Avec.

Big love to all of the fine folks at Adams Media for taking a chance on this book. I'm so honored and proud to be a part of your team.

Thanks to the contributors of this book. Actually, I'm not sure thanks will ever be enough. I am blessed to be in your company. You are all such talented writers and good friends.

I would be remiss if I didn't thank all of the teachers I've had over the years who encouraged me to write in the first place. Some of them are members of the cloth and no doubt my liberal use of the f-bomb has caused them to wonder where they went wrong. They are, in no particular order: the sisters at the Franciscan Learning Center in Joliet, Illinois; Sister Maria Goretti; Patricia Pierson; Patricia Yeager; Shelia Fry; William Bender; and Brother Tom Murphy, O.Carm.

Thanks and gratitude go to the editors with whom I worked during my time at the *Peoria Journal Star*, for being the firsts in a long line of editors to say, "This sucks. Go back and rewrite it." To Patricia B. Dailey who gave me a job I love getting up and going to every day.

To all of the readers of both ejshea.com and Lose the Buddha. Thank you so much for indulging me and my need to publish my drivel over the Internet. You all rock.

To Mindy Cohn, who took a little bit of a beating in this book but who was my hero growing up. Natalie *was* a writer after all. Blair may have gotten the boys, but she was never going to have a cool job.

Thanks to Chicago's Cheetah Gym, the Park District in Oak Brook, Illinois, and Weight Watchers for giving me the tools.

My friends are amazing and I'm lucky enough to have them in my life. Their support during this process kept me going. Thanks to the Diurna Girls; Wendy McClure; Jessamyn North; Candace Herr; Wesley MacMillan; Jacquelyn Lausch, Erin Azuse, and all of the Book Club girls; David Moll; Daniel Parenti; Steven Johnson; Jim and Wendy Becker; Jeanne Statts; Lora Sendag and Joy Evans. To Amy Janka who is living proof that goodness exists in the world and Allison Perlik without whom I'd be lost.

A special thanks goes to Pamela Ribon for doing it first, doing it best, and not minding my angsty e-mails during this process.

No one was ever so lucky as to be born or married into the family I was. To the Johnson/Mitchell/Atkins clans, especially Marceline O'Connor Johnson, for sharing Erik with me and for being my friend. To my grandmother, Kay Shea, for all she has taught me, the love she has shown me, and for the occasional, well-deserved eyebrow. To my aunt, Kathy Shea, for being my biggest cheerleader and for always, always, being there. To my sisters, Kendra Overstreet and Devyn Albritton, for helping me to learn who I am, and Kate Shea for being everything I ever hope to be. I love you, Schnooks. You are my heart.

To my parents, John and Lynette Shea. There will never be enough words to express my love and gratitude to you both. Lynette, you are both the reason I got through it and why I made peace with it all. I love you. Dad, you are my rock, my teacher, my confidant, my hero, and my friend.

Finally, and most importantly, to my husband, Erik Johnson: Erik offered me his shoulders to stand upon so I could see for the first time just how much beauty lay before me. Any of the good that I am is because of you, E. Thanks for all of the work *you* did in getting this book out. *Non mihi, non tibi, sed nobis.*

Contents

Introduction

EVERY FAT GIRL HAS COME TO THE POINT.

The Point, where she counts all of the pounds she could have lost had she not skipped that step class during week one, which led to drinking many beers on the Thursday of week two, which somehow begat week three's orgy of nachos, cupcakes, and meatball sandwiches. And she doesn't even like meatballs. The Point, when she thinks about the time she wasted eating anything not nailed securely to the table when she could have been working on losing weight.

She finds herself standing at the threshold of her dark kitchen. She is the picture of calm as she walks to the refrigerator, the voices in her head saying *don't, stop, you shouldn't.* She opens the door, comforted by the peaceful hum of the motor, the wedge of yellow light spills onto her face. Fervently, almost childlike, she reaches out for whatever she can as she whispers to herself:

"Monday. Monday is the day my diet starts."

"After this weekend I'll work out."

One day, I shut the refrigerator door.

Instead, I turned on my computer and began to write. I wrote about all of the hunger and aching and longing I felt at that moment. About the gym membership draining $60 of my paycheck on a monthly basis because I wasn't using it. I became obsessed with this process: I wrote about how constricting my pants were; how the pockets gave if I slumped back and let out my gut. I described how I could feel the mounds of flesh that shelved my breasts oozing over the top of my waistband, searching for somewhere to go.

I spent an agonizing evening dissecting my every feature, from my round face to my puzzling lack of torso. Then, I reached my legs. Strangely enough, I could find nothing wrong with them. Not a thing.

I pulled my leg up closer to my face so that I could closely inspect my thighs for doughy, pockmarked traces of fat and there was only smoothly pulled skin dusted with fine, blond wispy hairs. As I traveled farther down my leg, to the back of my knee, I saw only tendons and ocean-blue veins swimming about. Moving farther still, I reached my calf, thick with muscle that produced curved lines running parallel to each other and met, jutting out only at the bone of my ankle.

It was not the most perfect leg I had ever seen. But it was the first time I saw my leg and I didn't hate what was before me. More important, it was also the first time in my life I could see my entire body and what I'd been putting myself through. There I was, in my office, with my leg nearly wrapped around my head like a contortionist, arms flailing, my crotch hanging out in the wind. The next day, I got up and opened the refrigerator door. I made myself an egg-white omelet with red peppers and canned mushrooms. I strapped on my running shoes and walked to the park. I found a bench, sat back, and swung my leg completely over my head and held it there for three seconds.

When I got home, I e-mailed my friend Heather and asked her if she would design a weight-loss blog for me. I bought my ticket and packed my bags.

I found the way out of Big Girl Town.

This book is a collection of stories. It follows the journey of several women who got to The Point and found their own map out of Big Girl Town.

It is, as one of its writers is famous for saying, "diet-agnostic." Each writer has only two things in common: that she's lost weight and that as she boarded the bus out of town she chose to document her journey online for the world to read. We are all different shapes and sizes, different backgrounds and ages. Some of us have lost weight and kept it off. Some of us have hit a plateau and remained there. Some of us are still struggling. But we all have lived in Big Girl Town and we're not ashamed to talk about it.

For as delicious and decadent as being a resident of Big Girl Town can be, there is a seedy underbelly to it that few want to reveal.

There are sordid tales of pimps who go by the names of "Ben & Jerry" or "Cheetos" or, my personal favorite, "Super-Sized French Fries," dealing us the drugs we crave. There are the tourists, with their condescending "tsks," immediately followed with a "But you have such a pretty face!" reducing us to round, floating little heads bobbing around the planet trying not to make much noise or to be noticed at all for fear others might remind us of how much potential we're squandering because we're ordering a cheeseburger.

Because despite popular belief, no Fat Girl is ashamed of herself because of her weight until another person tells her she needs to be.

Weight loss takes hard work and examination of where we've been and where we are going. To ignore each other's stories is to ignore the problems that got us off that bus in the first place. But more than anything else, we know we're required to share our tales of gastronomic decadence because "Fat" is synonymous with "Bad."

Quite clearly, we've been bad. Oh, so very bad. And we've got quite a bit of explaining to do.

Within each other's words and stories we have found camaraderie among strangers whose experiences weren't so strange to us. Turns out, we were all neighbors in Big Girl Town. It took cyberspace to bring us together and learn that we weren't alone: The world is filled with women who are just like us.

We are the women of Big Girl Town. These are our stories.

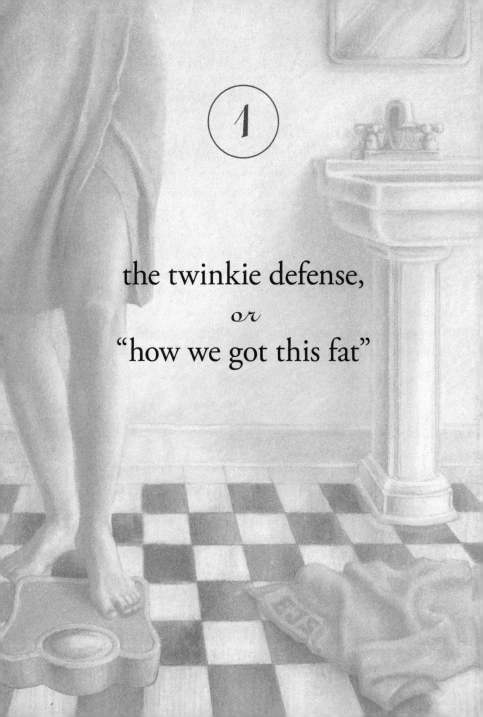

1

the twinkie defense,
or
"how we got this fat"

Fats

Beaming face. **Pink blouse with ruffled collar.** Big, crooked Chiclet teeth. My grade six photo shows a girl who is puffed up. In every sense of the word. Freshly permed hair. Teeth-strained lips. Cheeks by Pillsbury. And yes, a bit plucky and full of herself. Happy. Confident. Those were early days. Before the life-changing art assignment. It was simple enough. On one side of the construction paper, write in thick black marker, "I like:" On the other side, present a collage of images that illustrate what we indeed like, underscored by a written description. Do this three times. There was a stack of old magazines that we dove into in our quest to find things likeable. Once found, we hacked at them with safety scissors and pasted them onto our construction paper.

I think I was telling stories about my outrageous older sister who smoked funny-smelling cigarettes. The time flew. No time to reflect on what I liked. This called for some fast thinking.

So I grabbed a cooking magazine and with divine inspiration and the gross generalization that has plagued me my entire life, I cut out a mass of savory dishes and hurriedly pasted them onto my construction paper. It read:

I LIKE:
FOOD

By Susan Saundercook

Yep.

I like food. I can't remember the first two items on my list. But I can still see the grade six scrawl of letters spelling out *Food*. Mr. Phillips presented each piece of art. Shannon. She liked innocuous things like sports and dogs. Acceptable. Sherri liked skateboarding and dancing. Very cool. Then it was my turn. "Susan likes food."

At first there was a smattering of giggles. Then the class was awash with laughter. I was shocked. What the hell? Food. I should have been more specific like the other girls. I like candy. That was fine. I like chocolate. Great. "I like food." There was something gluttonous, foul, and excessive about that. My face burned. My eyes teared up. I couldn't believe this was happening.

And it happened over and over. I was called fats, hippo, pig, and cow all year. The boys would ask me, "What do you weigh?" And I'd answer cautiously, waiting for the punch line, "Eighty pounds?" And they'd have this look of glee before one of them spat out, "Yeah, eighty. On the *Richter* scale." That set the tone of the rest of the year. And in dramatic, weepy moments when I am watching "Confronting Former Bully" episodes on Ricki Lake, I am convinced it set the tone for my entire life to date. I never thought of myself as fat until that day. And now, no matter what my weight, I always think of myself as the Fat Girl who likes food.

How It's Done
By Julie Ridl

You don't just pop on 100 pounds. You don't just eat the pounds on in one sitting. It's rarely a matter of stuffing yourself silly. It's not very often a sudden or even creeping moral failure. It isn't about being lazy. It isn't any lack of discipline.

It's a subtle thing. It may begin early on with a lousy metabolism. Your brother may burn that 2,000 calories a day we keep hearing is common for healthy adults while you burn 1,200, or only 1,000 calories to get through your day. Some of us need to eat less than others, but we're all served the same sized portions. And if you're in a big family that competes over food, rewards with food, forces food, restricts food, you can become food-centric, liking it rather too much.

And now you're set up for it. Ready? You need only 1,200 calories a day, but you get 1,700. That's 500 calories too many. That's like a bagel with cream cheese too much. Or it's two bottles of pop too much. Within a week of overeating by that much, you've gained a pound. In a couple of months, you've put on 8 to 10 pounds. Your pants are tight. You decide to diet, making yourself hungry. You get tired of it and reward yourself the way you know how, with food. You have a bad day, you eat more. You rock up and down and up and down, and soon you just give in and get the bigger pants. They're not that much bigger.

You graduate from college, you fall in love, and you learn to cook. You taste things as you go, because you're serving somebody you care about and you want it to be right. So you get another 100 calories per meal more than you need. Maybe 200. Those extra calories bring the weight on faster. You gained 10 pounds this year.

Five of them just over the holidays.

You get ever more responsible jobs, because you're successful, even an overachiever. You work not forty hours a week, but fifty, maybe sixty, and maybe you're taking classes on top of that, raising a child. You have a few free hours each week, and you give those to your family, your community, your spouse, or your pets. You sure don't exercise anymore.

You either cook and eat or don't cook and eat terribly.

You get stressed, you eat.

You feel sad, you eat.

You are happy, you eat.

You win, you eat.

You lose, you eat.

You gain a pound or a half a pound a month, for a few years.

> You need only 1,200 calories a day, but you get 1,700. That's 500 calories too many. That's like a bagel with cream cheese too much.

You slowly lose touch with the way your body feels. Fat dulls your senses, insulates you from the world. If you got too much attention for your looks when you were younger, fat will turn down the volume. If people got too close, fat will put up a wall. If you are a woman in a man's world, fat will ease the tension, neuter you. You will be the jolly eunuch. You will be safe. Your spouse will not be jealous and your boss will not have to apologize to his wife for giving you a raise.

So you go on a diet. You lose most of the weight, or all of it. And finally, at last, you arrive at something close to the weight of your youth. Phew. You're done. You check weight-loss off your long to-do list. You go off your diet, stop working out.

And the next year you put it all back on and 10 pounds more.

And the next year you diet some off and put it on again. The net gain is 20 pounds. The year after that, 5. The year after that, 10.

And twenty years go by. You're forty years old, and you're 100, 120 pounds overweight.

It happens like that. It happens while you're behaving responsibly, working hard, contributing to your world, raising wonderful children, helping other people, contributing to charities, and paying only occasional attention to your body.

And then it all turns on you. Suddenly your joints can't take the strain. You hurt. You've gotten fat enough that now people think you lack discipline. You don't look good in the group photo. You look old. If you can't manage your weight, how can you manage that department? You are not paid as much as thinner people. You can't get a raise, a transfer, or a break. When you speak, you are not heard. In fact, people think all you do is whine.

> But your body, your miraculous body, responds. It responds slowly, surely, tentatively, sometimes reluctantly, but it does respond.

Your doctors don't take you seriously. Your family doesn't take you seriously. Your clients don't take you seriously. Because now your fat is in charge of the way people see you, hear you, believe you.

Your metabolism has shifted. Your body isn't responding to insulin now. You've dieted so well, so consistently, so successfully, that your low metabolism has lowered some more. And the diets stop working. You join Weight Watchers and GAIN weight.

The weight is coming on faster now, but you swear you're not eating much. You feel crazy. You are scared. Your feet swell up when you walk. Your hip gives out. You can't exercise enough to take the weight off and you can't eat any less without feeling sick and dizzy. You've tried every diet, every pill, every supplement. Everything.

Some days you call in sick and stay home under the covers.

And that's how it happens. And that's how it feels.

Working your way out of it takes serious medical help, a real leap of faith, and a determination to change your life completely. An overhaul.

It might mean quitting your job. I did.

It might mean giving up your cooking habit. I did that, too.

It might mean upsetting all the regular meal habits your family has established over the years, the holiday traditions. Cooking foods you've never tried, and eating a lot less of the ones you've relied upon for sustenance and comfort.

Did that and ditto.

You begin to move your body again, and you never stop.

That would be me.

And it takes a long time. But your body, your miraculous body, responds. It responds slowly, surely, tentatively, sometimes reluctantly, but it does respond. You learn things you didn't realize about the way it works. Like about that slow metabolism. About insulin and its effects. About how your body responds to food, about how food and emotions have gotten all mixed up over the years.

So much to learn and so much time to learn it.

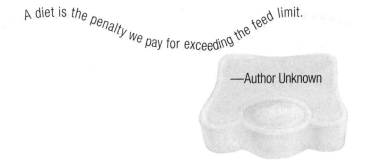

A diet is the penalty we pay for exceeding the feed limit.

—Author Unknown

Lessons Learned from Gym Class and the Starbuck's Drive-Through
By Heather Lockwood

I am sitting on the patio of a local Starbucks Coffee Shop just a few feet away from the drive-through. As I sit and ponder how I got fat, I am listening to order after order.

"Hi. Welcome to Starbucks. How can I help you?"
"I'll have a venti decaf mocha Frappuccino and a venti caramel Frappuccino."
"Would you like whip?"
"Yes, whip on both."
"That will be four fifty-nine. Please drive through."
"Hi. Welcome to Starbucks. How can I help you?"
"I would like an iced Frappuccino. Do you make those with skim?"
"We can."
"I'll have that with a chocolate, chocolate chip muffin."
"And what size is your Frappuccino?"
"Twenty ounces. Whatever that is."
"That will be five thirty-nine. Go ahead and drive through."

The orders continued:

"Venti iced caffè latte with vanilla."
"Venti mocha Frap with two shots of hazelnut with whip, no drizzle."

"Venti iced decaf latte."
"Grande caramel latte with soy and a grande vanilla Frappuccino."

8

And so on and so on and so on.

Once upon a time, I would have listened to these orders and thought, *Boy, does that sound good. In fact, that sounds great! How about I order myself one of those as well. And why not throw in a caramel fudge brownie, too? After all, I'm hungry.*

Now, things are different. I'm a born-again health fanatic and all I can think about while these people innocently order their beverages is, *Oooh. That's got to contain at least 600 calories.* Or, *Oh, man. Does she know she's about to consume the equivalent of a Big Mac Value meal?*

When I think about my former self and how I got fat, I want to plead ignorance. I contend my issues are the same as most of the American public. We have a problem with overeating and obesity. We live in a country where food is plentiful and cheap. We blindly order what sounds good to us with no thought of calories or fat. We fill our bodies with empty calories and are never the wiser for it. We go to McDonald's and Cinnabon and Denny's and the Cheesecake Factory and even Starbucks, where we are loaded with calorie-packed sustenance that our bodies don't stand a chance of burning. And we don't even realize what we are doing. Or we do and we just don't care.

As a recovering mindless eater, I now suffer from the affliction of overedification. I can't help but listen and assess every order I hear given and every grocery cart I see full. I do this because I was there. I was in that place where I'd eat a sackful of French fries and a medium chocolate shake for lunch, not just because it tasted good, but because it was easy and just around the corner from my work. I had no concept of balance. I wouldn't have known a square meal if it had dropped on my head.

No one taught me the rules of nutrition. No one taught me about portion sizes. I had to seek this information for myself. My childhood experience with eating was quite the contrary. I lived off sugar-filled

Flintstones Vitamins (which I would steal if the occasion presented itself) and pudding in a can. We had Little Debbie Oatmeal Sandwiches as a snack after school. I drank chocolate milk by the gallon. One of my favorite games was the one where I'd sit on the kitchen counter after mixing a glass of milk with a spoonful of Nestle Quik. I would then proceed to drink the chocolate concoction spoonful by spoonful telling myself it was medicine. "Just what the doctor ordered."

I learned early on that food was comfort. Food was security. We celebrated my chorus recitals with a trip to the Dairy Queen. Going to Grandma's meant I'd be greeted at the door with hot buttered toast. When I was stuck in my father's office late at night as he was finishing up his work, I got the consolation prize of a trip to the vending machine, where the decision was a tough one: a Snickers or a Hostess Cherry Pie.

Occasionally there was a night when I had to eat Brussels sprouts or a bowl of spinach. But I was never taught about limits or portion sizes. Nutrition was just an afterthought. Being full and satiated was the primary goal.

> I learned early on that food was comfort. Food was security.

While I learned poor eating habits and gained weight as a child, I wasn't all that low on self-esteem. I guess you could say my momma raised me right. I'd play dress-up when everyone was out of the house. I'd put on an old tube-top that came from Lord-knows-where. I'd steal a pair of high heels from my mother's closet. I'd take an old cigarette butt out of an ashtray and watch myself in the bathroom mirror practicing, "Tell me about it, Stud."

"Tell *me* about it, Stud."

"*Tell* me about it, Stuuuud."

I wanted to be Olivia Newton-John from *Grease*. It didn't matter that, at ten, my face was already rounder than hers. It didn't matter that baby fat squeezed out from under and above the tube top. Those things

10

weren't clear to me in the mirror looking out. I didn't see a fat child. I just saw an attractive girl dreaming of what she wanted to be.

Even though I weighed more than my friends, I knew I still had "a pretty face." I lived for that line. I gained confidence from that line. Staring into that same mirror, I'd look at my eyes and acknowledge how pretty they were. I'd play with my hair and tell myself, *I'm pretty*.

So, no, self-esteem wasn't really an issue.

At least, it wasn't an issue until junior high. Once in seventh grade, the weight differences became noticeable. While I was buying women's size 11, my girlfriends wore sizes 6 and 8. In the locker room before gym, I could see the sizes staring out from their clothing. I was envious. I wanted to be like them. This was one of the first signs I was not. I was different.

Those moments in gym were always the most painful not just because of the locker room. They were also painful because my lack of fitness and coordination made all of my inadequacies stand out. The ten-minute run was the gym activity I dreaded the most. My girlfriends didn't like it either, but they completed it fine. They would run the entire thing and even be able to talk afterward. But I was always the one at the very end with the obese kids and misfits. My skin would turn a nasty reddish color and I'd be gasping for air. In very desperate situations, I'd even stop and walk a bit until the gym teacher would tell me to pick it up.

There was volleyball, too. I couldn't bump, set, or spike, and I was always picked last for teams. When I was on the court, I remember the girls would cover me in what I thought at the time was kindness. Now I realize they didn't want me to get my hands on the ball any more than I did since they were sure I would just knock the thing out of bounds.

Those forty-five minutes of gym class were always the longest and most dreaded of the day throughout my entire school experience. Out of my gym clothes, my insecurities disappeared. I knew I was a smart kid. I knew I was a pretty kid. So what if I couldn't bump, set, or spike?

Where would that get me?

Any gym-related inadequacies were made up for with good grades and overparticipation in school activities. I was on the yearbook staff, in the choir, and show choir. I performed in plays, wrote for the newspaper, and competed on the speech team. Every teacher in the school loved me and I basked in the glow of their praise. My self-esteem was higher than ever. It didn't matter that I wore the same jean size as my mom. I was a grade-A student. I had a beautiful voice. I had a pretty face.

Now cut to fifteen years later and here I am at thirty-two, and I am obsessed with nutrition. I am obsessed with what the media calls the "crisis of obesity in our country." Even more, I am training for a half-marathon. The ten-minute run I used to dread is now just a warm-up for me. And even though, to this day, I lack good hand-eye coordination and wouldn't set foot near a volleyball court, activity and the gym are an important part of my life.

The truth is, the inactivity of my childhood and adolescence caught up with me. I could no longer ignore the size discrepancy between my peers and myself. I could no longer ignore my poor diet. And I was no longer satisfied with my less-than-physical accomplishments. My body deserved better.

This revelation hit me the hardest on a day hike with some friends. By this time I was at my highest weight ever. I was happily married. My husband and I were active and social. But my eating was out of control. And my activity level was at an all-time low. Yet, when a couple of friends invited us hiking, I didn't even dream that my physical state would become an issue.

But it did.

I was carrying an extra 30 pounds of weight and facing a half-mile climb up to the top of a bluff at Devil's Lake Park in Baraboo, Wisconsin. It was a beautiful fall day. The sun was shining. The air was crisp.

And as my buddies and my husband climbed, my heart rate started to soar. Sweat was escaping from every pore within minutes. I watched my companions move farther and farther out of my sight and I knew I had no other choice but to stop and rest. I was only a quarter of the way into the hike and I just couldn't take it. I had to stop every ten or so steps. Soon our friends were completely out of sight. Soon my husband was climbing back down to join me after realizing I had fallen behind. And there he waited with me each time I had to take a breath, each time I had to steady my feet, each time I had to take a drink of water and curse the sun and rocks and circumstances that had led me to that point.

> Living to be old and healthy is all the argument I need when I consider skipping the gym or ordering that venti Frappuccino with whip.

When I reached the top of the bluff, my friends were relaxing in the shade. "Really, it's no problem. We didn't mind waiting" was all they said. But I was humiliated. I felt gross and out of shape and unworthy. Most of all, I was sad. How could a twenty-five-year-old be this badly out of shape? Even worse, I wondered what would happen to me later. How would this body handle another twenty-five years?

That was the turning point, really. From that hike on, I vowed to exercise more regularly. I tested my progress each fall with a climb up that very same bluff. The first time I made it up the entire way without stopping, I knew I had turned a corner. Life would never be the same. Activity and nutrition needed to be part of my life if I wanted to live to be old and healthy.

Living to be old and healthy. Now that is a concept. Now that is a reason to change bad lifestyle habits. Living to be old and healthy is all the argument I need when I consider skipping the gym or ordering that venti Frappuccino with whip. Sometimes I think of myself as

enlightened. It is hard not to sitting next to the drive-through at a Starbucks Coffee Shop. But the truth is, I'm just well educated. I won't lie;
the education was hard won. I had to do it myself.

I had a great childhood. I wouldn't trade those hours spent imitat-
ing Olivia in front of the bathroom mirror for a million dollars. But I do
wish that I could have learned a little earlier on what health and well-
ness was all about. I wish someone could have shown me that gym class
wasn't necessarily all that scary. Those are things that I did miss out on
in my youth. I won't make that same mistake with my own children.
Frappuccinos are for special occasions. Broccoli, on the other hand, is
for every day.

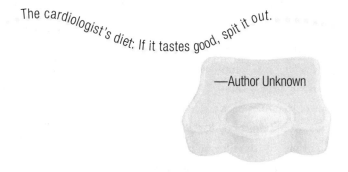

The cardiologist's diet: If it tastes good, spit it out.

—Author Unknown

Endless Celery
By Shauna Marsh

I was born the poor child of a Weight Watchers leader. Well, we weren't particularly poor, but the Weight Watchers thing is true.

I didn't start out a fat child, but I was sure exposed to a lot of it. Every Monday night my sister and I tagged along to Mum's class. We were supposed to play quietly in a corner, but I found it all too fascinating. The women would queue up week after week, their eyes full of fear or weariness or both, handing over a handsome sum of money to step on a scale and be told if they'd been good or bad.

Afterward, they'd sit in a circle of clunky metal chairs, confessing their sins or squawking about their success. I listened carefully as they discussed how brown bread was good and ice cream was bad—unless it was Weight Watchers' own brand, of course. I learned one could eat endless celery and lettuce, but the world would collapse if you had more than two eggs per week. I took in all this information and began to realize that weight was a really big deal.

One night at Weight Watchers, I sneaked onto the scale. It said 85 pounds. I don't know if that was overweight for a kid, but I certainly looked okay. Even then I was getting taller. But the weigh-lady popped up behind me and peered at the number. She spoke to my mother like I wasn't even there. "My god! She's big! She nearly weighs as much as I do!"

This woman was only 4'10" and tiny as can be. But of course, I went home and cried. From that moment on, I saw myself as a horrible fat person.

Food for me was always divided into good and evil. As a Weight Watchers leader, my mother always cooked healthy meals. We rarely had chocolate or ice cream in the house; we never had butter on our sandwiches or cookies with our lunch. It was commendable that she brought us up knowing how to eat well, but it always left me with this screwy attitude about food. Whenever I went to my dad's house on a weekend, I'd scoff into his white bread and chocolate biscuits, feeling so very guilty and euphoric, knowing I'd eaten something bad.

I dieted on and off right through high school. When puberty kicked in I was a size 10, and bigger and taller than my friends, which added to that freakish feeling. It didn't help when both my father and stepfather would make idle comments like, "You'd be so pretty if you just lost a little bit of weight." My friends were baffled when I refused to eat pizza and candy at slumber parties. Their parents would tell me to eat up; I was a great kid with no reason to be so obsessed about food.

I wrote in my diary at fifteen, rather melodramatically but heartfelt nonetheless, "I'm 130 pounds and I want to die."

But I knew I was fat. My family told me so, and family knows best, right? I'd look in the mirror and get angry at my reflection. I wrote in my diary at fifteen, rather melodramatically but heartfelt nonetheless, "I'm 130 pounds and I want to die."

I stopped going swimming after a family holiday. We were on the beach and I was parading around in my new swimsuit when my mother casually said, "You have a nice shape you know, if you could just make it a little smaller." I replayed that comment over and over in my head. I started to avoid clothes that showed off my body. I made excuses to not go to parties. If a boy looked at me and smiled, I'd turn away and think he was mocking me. I was invited to go on a school exchange to Japan for a year, but I turned it down because I thought I was too fat to go and I wouldn't be accepted.

It wasn't until the eleventh grade when I started to *really* get fat.

Our Weight Watchers meeting closed down because the leader was very uninspiring and everyone had stopped coming. At the same time, I started working part-time at a fast-food joint. That's when I started to lose my way.

The more stressful school got, the more withdrawn I became. I turned to food as a diversion. My minimum wage finally gave me the means to indulge in all the forbidden foods on my mother's list. I'd buy chocolate bars and scoff them down under the covers at night. I'd stuff the wrappers under my mattress, then cry myself to sleep. I used to sneak greasy food at work whenever I had a chance. As soon as I was alone, I ate. It felt so wrong but somehow exhilarating at the same time.

When I finished high school I weighed 220 pounds. I moved out of home for university. At first I made an attempt to buy healthy food and lost a few pounds, but then I went into another phase of food rebellion. Now that Mum wasn't looking, I gorged on chocolate, chips, ice cream, and takeout food.

My weight soared. In the three years of college, I put on almost 70 pounds. For a while I kidded myself that I could "carry it off"—being 5'8" I could attribute a fair amount of weight as "curves." But soon I lost any shapeliness. My waist soon blended with my boobs, and my stomach had three tiers like a big fat wedding cake.

Whether I consciously realized it or not, soon my life was dictated by my weight. After I finished my degree, I was confused about my career path and my bulk was a convenient distraction. I made half-hearted attempts to find a real job, but I was so ashamed of my size that I was convinced no one would employ me. To make it worse, I worked in a greasy spoon, and soon all the fries and burgers added to my bulk.

My boss was also overweight. She joined Weight Watchers and had bombed out after ten weeks, but told me it was great these days with the POINTS system, so why don't I try it? I did. I was gobsmacked when

17

I weighed in at 293 pounds. On the way home I bought McDonald's for dinner and cried into my fries.

I stayed for nine weeks, losing 13 pounds, but my heart wasn't in it. By then I was so depressed that I would spend all day lying on the floor crying, or looking at the mirror in disgust, pounding it with my fists and sobbing. I couldn't sleep; my head was so foggy I couldn't think.

Finally one day my mother called and she ask chirpily, "How are you doing?" and I broke down, told her I was falling apart. I was never suicidal; I didn't have the energy to harm myself.

I got help. I went along to a counselor and uncovered a lot of painful stuff. But my denial was so strong that I somehow managed not to attribute any of it to my weight.

I started taking antidepressants and quit Weight Watchers. In the end I opted for a complete change, moving interstate and pursuing a completely different career path.

Two years passed. I focused on getting my act together. I moved to a new city, earned a graphic design diploma, and got a fantastic job. On the surface it seemed like I'd completely transformed myself. I'd even managed to kick the antidepressants and convinced myself I felt balanced and happy.

I was so caught up in my new life that I didn't pause to think about my skyrocketing weight. I continued to binge and ignored the fact I was buying a bigger size every time I went clothes shopping. By the end of 2000 I could barely squeeze into a size 28. I kept myself busy with work so I didn't have any time to notice that I didn't have a life to speak of, that I never went out to clubs, had boyfriends, or went on vacation.

I'd convinced myself that this was how my life was meant to be. I'd built myself a big blubber fortress to hide behind, so I'd never have to do anything scary in life. But something had to change—after all, there was nothing bigger in the shops than a size 28.

To Scratch an Itch
By Erin J. Shea

very person who is overweight has to have some sort of story as to how he or she ended up fat in the first place.

It's almost as if in order for the earth to continue spinning on its axis, there has to be a reason and a justification for the fat. The fat can't just be fat, as it exists on the person's body. The fat has to be symbolic of the human condition. Perhaps a tortured love affair, 2.5 kids and a picket fence, a childhood spent unloved and ignored, a stressful life, or at the very least, a cruel joke played by God wherein its bearer has a genetic predisposition to inhale all food within his or her path.

For people to accept the story of a fat person, there has to be, in fact, a *good* story. Don't tell anyone that the pounds just "crept up on you"—as if one fine day during college those thunder thighs of yours jumped out from the shadows like two meaty, cellulite-filled assailants and landed on your once-perfect body.

Nobody likes that story and they sure as hell aren't going to believe you if you tell it.

They want to know about those days after school when you got off the bus and headed straight for the refrigerator, toasted four slices of white bread to a perfect shade of brown, slathered each with a thick layer of Miracle Whip, and devoured them one by one during the latest episode of *Degrassi Junior High*.

What everyone wants to hear about is the pompom coach from high school who pulled you aside and told all 115 pounds of you that while you were a great dancer and had the routine down solid, what kept you from making the squad was your weight.

19

They want to know of those nights you spent broke and alone in that first apartment of yours, reading Oprah's account about how at her rock bottom she gorged on half-frozen hot dog buns dressed in maple syrup. They want to know how at that moment you wondered to yourself if you had any hamburger buns left over from last weekend's barbeque.

Those are the stories that count. Those are the ones that make sense. And while fat is generally arbitrary in terms of perception, most everyone has their very own mayo, pompom, or glutton-filled, depression-soaked story.

This is mine.

There wasn't a moment in my life that I wasn't aware that I was overweight. I knew I was Irish. I knew I was Italian. I knew that I had brown hair that fell past my shoulders in wavy strands. I knew my eyes were blue and that my skin was so pale that if the sun shone down upon me you could see the thin, blue veins taking up residence underneath.

I knew I was fat. Knowing was really that simple; it was an undeniable element of my physical makeup.

I have my share of depressing stories wherein I calmed myself by eating, aggravating my situation. At eleven, immediately after my parents' divorce but before my father remarried, I blocked out my mother's screaming by slamming back cans of salad croutons and washing them down with peanut butter cups. There was the two years after that, when my dad was out of a job, now supporting a family with four children instead of two. My grade school's yearly fundraiser was fast approaching. Each student was charged with selling $50 worth of $1 candy, a task that would have been easy had I not had to compete for customers with my three sisters.

I brought home my supply and proceeded to eat $25 worth of caramel and crisped-rice-filled chocolate bars before I knew what hit me.

I numbed myself with enough sugar that the fear I previously felt was only an abstract concept. The only feeling that remained was that of the gobs of melted chocolate dripping from my lips.

I have more stories like these, though gorging on too many of these sad Fat Girl stories is as self-indulgent as eating an entire pan of pasta carbonara in one sitting—it's just fine going down but too much leaves you bloated. Besides, for as many sad Fat Girl stories as I have, there are just as many that offer up no emotional connection to my weight problem whatsoever.

At the end of the day, my childhood traumas and the coping mechanisms I developed as a result didn't help matters much. On the occasion that I am stressed or anxious I still head for the cupboards like I'm on autopilot. Though at twenty-nine years old, I find it difficult to blame my parents' divorce for why I'm wolfing down Cheetos like it's my job and I'm gunning for a promotion. Doing so always seemed like a cliché, a reason given all too often, an excuse whose validity has run its course for me.

> I have more stories like these, though gorging on too many of these sad Fat Girl stories is as self-indulgent as eating an entire pan of pasta carbonara in one sitting . . .

I eat because I like to eat. Food is a religion for me, a way of life. I am obsessed with food—how it is prepared, how it is presented, and how it tastes. The manifestation of food in its most beautiful and artistic form is awe-inspiring. Most of us still gather as a community when food is the focus. Little else excites me as much as an evening spent around my parents' table enjoying the latest creation to spring forth from their kitchen. There is always laughter and joy. The meal itself is a cause for celebration as much as is our coming together as a family.

My love of food is so great that I currently make my living writing about food, specifically the restaurant industry. The majority of my day is spent understanding the latest food trends and interviewing the operators and owners of the very places that have served as my churches since I was a little girl.

And the more years that pass by, the more adverse I am to buying in to the notion that food is bad. That food, in fact, is something to fear. Global warming is something to fear. Losing your job is something to fear. Having your leg shorn off by an errant buzz saw is something to fear. I've yet to see any conclusive evidence to prove to me that a hamburger or two is going to do as much damage as any of these things could. I suppose it is my distaste for treating food like it is an instrument of the devil, and subsequently the culture perpetuating this idea, that accounts for my weight problems as an adult.

At twenty-nine years old, I find it difficult to blame my parents' divorce for why I'm wolfing down Cheetos like it's my job and I'm gunning for a promotion.

You mean I'm really less of a person because I'm eating this slice of cake? Explain to me how if I decide to eat a bowl of potato chips, this behavior means I possess little to no self-esteem. How is it that I am doomed to an eternity filled with no one to love me and a sadness the likes of which humankind has never known if I order the crab Rangoon from my favorite Chinese carryout joint?

Defiantly, I have eaten all of these things and then some as my own personal "Fuck You" to a society that has repeatedly told me that I'm required to handle every morsel in front of me with kid gloves. Sure, I've spent more than my share of time laying blame for my myriad problems squarely at the foot of the very altar of the food that I worship, but the majority of my adult life has been spent treating it with the sort of reverence found in monasteries.

The flip side to my little anarchist bent is that such unadulterated avarice without consequence is only afforded to those born with the metabolism of a jackrabbit in heat. I am not one of those people. Embracing food and thumbing my nose at the Fat Girl stereotype has turned me into a Fat Girl.

Three years ago, I woke up in the middle of the night to scratch an itch I had lurking on my right upper thigh. I was lying on my right side and I moved my left hand downward to relieve the itch when something odd happened. I couldn't get to my thigh without first moving my gut out of the way. My stomach actually thwarted the simple act of scratching an itch. I was somewhere around 188 pounds and while I suffered no serious emotional problems as a result, I knew something had to give.

For the first time, I knew I had to find some peace with the food that I loved and the fat that was a consequence of my devotion without hating myself or reverting to type.

Food isn't bad and I'm not a bad person for enjoying it so much. As a result of eating too much food and not expending the energy it takes to burn off the excess, the only thing I am is fat.

And I just don't want to be fat anymore.

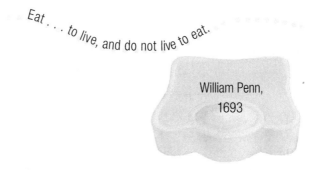

Eat . . . to live, and do not live to eat.

William Penn,
1693

Food, Glorious Food
By Robyn Anderson

$\mathcal{I}$'ve always been fat.

I say that, but I have a picture of myself at the age of six, wearing a pink bikini and running on the beach, not fat by any stretch of the imagination. I remember feeling fat already at that point in my life, though. My mother walked every day for exercise when we lived in Guam (I was an Air Force brat), and I remember one day running up to her with a friend and saying, "Suzanne and I ran around the *whole* block and didn't stop even once!" and my mother saying with great pleasure, "Good!"

Well. Except that Suzanne and I had really more *moseyed* around the block than ran it, stopping to dip our hands in a lawn sprinkler and wiping our faces with water so that it would look like we'd been sweating profusely. I suspect that my mother wasn't taken in by my wily ruse, but she pretended well enough, and I went away from the encounter believing she was snowed.

At some point after I was six and before I was nine, I started to gain weight. I have a picture of myself at the age of nine, a big fake smile plastered on my round face and a thickening layer of fat on my belly. I had my father take my picture because I'd read in *Teen Beat* that when you write a fan letter to a celebrity, they really like it if you include a picture of yourself. Later that year, I wrote a letter to Marie Osmond and enclosed that picture, begging her to help me with my weight. I had read that she weighed 98 pounds soaking wet, and I had a vision of her swooping down like a fairy godmother and whisking me off to Osmondland, where she would teach me how to smile that Osmond smile, how to stay rail-thin, and in no time flat I'd be slipping into the clothes the skinny girls in my class wore.

Also, Donny Osmond would take one look at me and fall in love. Convert to Mormonism? Anything for you, Donny.

There wasn't a lot of junk food in our house while I was growing up. We often had dessert, but once the dessert had been served, any leftovers were put away and not available to us kids.

I think it's fair to say that with age came autonomy, and with that came the ability to buy and eat loads of junk food that my mother knew nothing about, eating in secret in my room when I was sure no one would barge in. When I was six, my mother yelled at my sister and me for eating Kool-Aid mix straight from the packet at a neighbor's house. We were amazed that she knew what we'd been doing; I'm sure our big purple-stained lips had nothing to do with her figuring it out. At nine I was allowed to ride my bike across the Air Force base to the store where I—unbeknownst to my parents—bought ice cream and candy bars. When I was thirteen I rode my bike to the neighborhood store and loaded up on doughnuts. The more freedom I had, the more junk food I was able to buy and eat, and the more weight I gained. There were diets along the way, but by the time I was seventeen and had my driver's license and a part-time job at McDonald's, I weighed more than 200 pounds. I remember my amazement the first time I stepped on the scale and saw 204.

But I wasn't amazed enough to do anything about it.

I stayed somewhere between 200 and 225 pounds for the next two years, but I ate more and more in secret: in the car, in my room, eating

> When I was six, my mother yelled at my sister and me for eating Kool-Aid mix straight from the packet at a neighbor's house.

quickly and then chewing gum or breath mints to cover the smell of sugary food on my breath. When I got pregnant at the age of nineteen, I weighed about 225. I took the idea of "eating for two" to heart. My then-husband and I moved from a small apartment with a loft bedroom to a slightly larger two-bedroom apartment, located directly behind a Dairy Queen. You can imagine how many hot fudge sundaes I ate over the course of the next six months. He ate along with me, matching me bite for bite, and never gained an ounce. The bastard.

The day I went into the hospital to have my daughter delivered by cesarean section, I weighed 275 pounds. Rather than requiring me to move my hugely pregnant body out to the nurse's station so I could be weighed—I'm sure the sight of my ass hanging out the back of the jonny would have scared anyone into hard labor—the nurse asked me how much I weighed. I looked pointedly at my mother and then-husband sitting across the room from my hospital bed. My mother laughed, rolled her eyes, and covered her ears.

"One seventy-five. Uh, I mean, two seventy-five," I said.

When my mother uncovered her ears, my then-husband told her how much I weighed.

My daughter only weighed 10 pounds and 2 ounces, so unfortunately, I couldn't blame the whole 50-pound gain on her. I lost a lot of weight right after I had her, getting back down to the 220s—I was young and clueless and doing well to get her fed, let alone myself—but that weight came back eventually, and as is usually the case when rebound weight hits, I gained a lot more as well.

Between the ages of twenty and twenty-eight, my weight went up to and past 300 pounds. *Three hundred pounds*. I was horrified to see that number on the scale, but I wasn't as surprised as I'd been when I hit 200 at seventeen.

When I was twenty-eight, I divorced my first husband. When I met the man who would become my second husband, Fred, I hovered around 300 pounds. We moved in together and ate and ate and ate. After we'd been together for two and a half years, we got married. We celebrated our marriage by grilling shrimp and steaks and eating cake and Halloween candy. We got married on Halloween so that Fred would always remember our anniversary.

As married life went on, we continued to eat. And then one day I stepped on the scale to find that it could only weigh up to 350 pounds and I was more than that. I eventually discovered that I weighed 362 pounds.

I was 362 pounds, and gunning for 400.

Finally enough to stop me in my tracks.

> Inside some of us is a thin person struggling to get out, but they can usually be sedated with a few pieces of chocolate cake.
>
> —Author Unknown

End Zone
By Lori Ford

When I was eight, my grandparents took me to visit Busch Gardens in Tampa. According to the story, it seemed all I wanted to do was eat. Every time I'd eat an ice cream, I'd ask for another one, or cotton candy, or candy apple, or candy, or whatever I saw. It was constant—me asking for more junk food. They even forced me to eat a healthy meal, but it had no effect. Immediately upon completion, I asked for dessert.

By the end of the day, they called my mother back at home, completely annoyed by my behavior.

The day began with a stupendous, happy vacation breakfast of blueberry pancakes, and then my grandmother suggested a chocolate ice cream for a midmorning snack; then I saw something else, asked for it, and got it—and it was all over. I wanted everything.

I'm sure at some point someone said, "Listen here, missy. You've eaten quite enough," and I turned beet red from embarrassment and craved another ice cream cone to relax my anxious state. I may have even asked for it, which led to the phone call.

My mom always had me on a diet, and no doubt she was angry to learn I'd blown my very strict diet to pieces while on vacation. She would be pissy the moment I got off the plane and she would tell me how puffy I looked and not want to talk to me. This, of course, would make me anxious and therefore hungry, and I'd have to sit there fighting with myself the whole ride home over whether to ask her for something to eat.

And maybe that is what I always do, and every time I get a boyfriend and the excitement feels like an amusement park vacation, I find myself unable to turn down any of the foods I know I'm not supposed to eat. Then one treat leads to another and another, and next thing you know I'm puffy and wondering why he no longer seems attracted to me. Then I feel anxious and want to sneak stuff. Next thing you know, I can't wear my clothes. Once a hottie in a slip dress, I'm now sporting track-suits with chocolate stains.

I've struggled with my weight my whole life. I'm struggling today and I'll be struggling tomorrow. This is regardless of whether I eat a brownie today or not. A brownie is a thirty-second break from a lifetime struggle. I've gained because I'm tired of the daily fight with myself to count every calorie and exercise. I've gained because right now I don't feel like I can count calories for the rest of my life, so I really don't want to do it today, either. I've gained because if anything is offered to me at any point of the day I will say yes, and then whatever I've done all day to make it a first "good day" will be over and I'll be headed toward my next pound gained. Every time I've ever lost weight, I was in "the zone." This occurs when I get so angry, so frustrated, so tired of being fat that a light goes off and a great wind blows past my face and next thing you know I'm un-freaking-stoppable. I'm currently not in the zone. I beg for the zone. I plead for the zone. I wake up every day and feel around to see if it's there. It's not there.

> Once a hottie in a slip dress, I'm now sporting tracksuits with chocolate stains.

The zone is a wonderfully calm place to be. It's like I'm surrounded by an invisible force field that protects me from stress. My determination is so strong, I never doubt myself. If I see a bad number on the scale, it makes me more determined not less. Somewhere around goal weight, the zone fades, slightly at first. Then I feel hungrier and give in a little more often since my clothes fit and I feel great. Then, my desire for desserts grows stronger and stronger. I want desserts every night. I can't imagine a life without desserts. I have the desserts, but my desire doesn't stop there. No, it gets worse and I want treats all the time. Next thing you know, I'm out of the zone. It happens with Chinese food and pizza, too. They're all my trigger foods.

When my weight starts creeping up, at first I think it's no big deal. I can knock off 5 pounds, no problem. But instead, I learn to accept the 5 pounds. It doesn't affect my clothing size. I still feel sexy, so what's the harm? Then I'm up 10 pounds. Some clothes start getting tight, but I pretend I don't want to wear them anyway. They are my super-skinny clothes. I was foolish for buying them. Who could stay such a small size? I convince myself that maintaining would be too difficult and I'd be hungry all the time. Besides, I still feel great. There are plenty of adorable clothes left to wear.

Twenty pounds later, I know I've got a problem. I'm more self-conscious about my body. My clothes either don't fit well or stop fitting. I really hunker down at this point and give a good effort to diet it off. Either I'm successful, and I have been many times, or I start dieting and failing, giving up and restarting. I feel out of control and frustrated, and in my frustration, I often turn to food. I can gain another 10, 20, 50 pounds at this point. It's a very sad and scary place to be. And I'm there right now.

I've struggled with my weight my whole life. I'm struggling today and I'll be struggling tomorrow.

I have such high hopes. I wake up ready to start the day. Heck, I even get on the scale to have a proper "before" weight. Driving to work I'm already thinking about food, about how breakfast is the most important meal of the day and you aren't supposed to skip breakfast and how it jump-starts your metabolism for the day and how I don't have time to stop at Hardees, but I could have Oreos from the vending machine. I'm hungry by 10 A.M. and by 11 A.M. it takes every bit of energy not to eat a snack. Lunch finally arrives and I can barely contain myself. I eat out and spend about half a day's worth of calories. By 2 P.M. I'm hungry again and have to occupy my mind for the next three hours. Sometimes I make it, sometimes I don't. If something stressful happens during this period, I most likely break. If I can stuff down my hunger and make it until I get home, only then do I have something to eat. Sadly, I know at this point that a 1,200-calorie day is impossible. A snack-size amount of calories won't hold me until dinner and dinner is so late I'm famished again and can't stop myself from overeating. I'm also miserable about the whole experience at this point, so if ice cream or something delectable is offered, there's no way I'm turning it down.

I've been trying to shake up the routine. I bring something healthy to work, like an egg omelet. I have string cheese for a snack. These foods are supposed to help my hunger, but I still crave chocolate and I'm still just as hungry by lunch as if I didn't eat at all. I can't seem to cut my lunch calories because they don't even last me until dinner as it is. I'm trying to remember how the heck I managed to do this before. I remember that after a few days the hunger becomes a dull ache. It's there but it's manageable. It may take a hot bath to get away from the kitchen or going to bed sometimes at 7 P.M., but it is manageable. Certainly I can live this way the rest of my life. Certainly hunger becomes a distant thought. If it really is hunger.

I try to think about what I'm going through. Am I bored, am I wishing for more out of life? Something is still missing and if I could fill that void, perhaps I wouldn't be hungry anymore. But I haven't a clue what it is. And it's something that chocolate would take care of *right now*.

Nothing Ventured, Nothing Lost
By Monique van den Berg

Here's my theory: Thin people who become fat are different from people who have always struggled with their weight.

I'm not sure if it's harder for them, the once-thin, or if it's easier. On the one hand, if they know what it is to be a thin adult, maybe it's harder to deal with being fat. Maybe they're more critical of themselves; the self-esteem so crucial to weight loss is harder for them to come by.

But on the other hand, maybe it's easier for them to get thin again, because they *think* of themselves as thin, each one defining herself as "a thin person." There is a fundamental psychological hurdle they don't need to jump. That strikes me as quite an advantage.

Because I, on the other hand, can't even imagine what it's like to be thin. I was an overweight kid and I'm an overweight adult. And—possibly the most crucial distinction of all—I've always thought of myself as fat.

Of course, I've dieted. Ever since I was a kid and my mother put me on the ridiculous string bean diet. But as an adult, I never wanted to *admit* that I was dieting. Admitting that I was dieting would be admitting that I was fat, and I was sort of hoping nobody would notice.

I halfheartedly tried dieting over the years, but there was too much shame involved in taking it seriously. I was afraid I would fail. Whereas if I didn't try at all, there could be no failure. And of course, I was basically a happy, healthy person. I was just a happy, healthy size 24 and I was getting bigger, not smaller. And every extra pound made me a little less happy, a little less healthy.

I was happier after I moved to San Francisco and took up bike riding and subsequently lost some weight. In fact, I dropped down to a size

18 (a plus-size 18) without changing my eating habits at all. And I felt sexier, healthier, and better. I was thrilled with my new body, although by the standards of the Paris Hiltons of the world, I was still an enormous cow. (Then again, to the Paris Hiltons of the world, anyone over a size 2 is an enormous cow.)

Once my schedule got too busy for regular bike riding, the weight began creeping back up again. And it was at that moment that I began to panic. I didn't want to go back into the twenties. I liked being a size 18.

At the same time, a good friend of mine had joined Weight Watchers. She was hipper than me, more dedicated than me, cooler than me in every way—and she wasn't ashamed to say, "Yep, I'm doing this." Her success (more than 90 pounds lost) and her attitude inspired me to join Weight Watchers with her. And it was much easier than I thought it would be—not the program itself, but admitting I was doing it in the first place.

> I am still, in my own head, a Fat Girl. A Fat Girl who can do all these things—a Fat Girl who feels fabulous about herself—but a Fat Girl nonetheless.

Walking through the door and stepping on the scale, I faced up to the number: 263. It was my failures and weaknesses quantified, that number. And that was my challenge: somehow, with grace, to leave the number 263 behind me for good.

I lost 50 pounds in a year, with more to go, and then stalled. Or looked at another way, I lost 50 pounds and kept it off. My friend and I were both overweight, but she lost it far more quickly than I did. Is it because she was a thin person who had gained weight, whereas I was a fat person who was simply getting fatter, adjusting the exact degree of fatness? Maybe. Probably.

I know that I still have weight to lose, both physical and psychological weight. But I've experienced the rewards of losing weight. I get compliments from people who haven't seen me in a long time. I can ride on the back of a motorcycle. I can shop at clothing stores other than Lane Bryant. I can wear a tiny black dress with confidence, in front of my ex-boyfriends. I can walk farther and faster. I am stronger.

But I am still, in my own head, a Fat Girl. A Fat Girl who can do all these things—a Fat Girl who feels fabulous about herself—but a Fat Girl nonetheless.

That Fat Girl has done some amazing things. Sure she's resented her thin friends, outgrown her pants, and binged on doughnuts, but she's also gotten me where I am today. It was that Fat Girl who lost those 50 pounds. She was the one who walked into Weight Watchers and decided to make a change. She was the one who ate salads instead of cheeseburgers. And I wonder if there's a good chance that, no matter how much weight I lose, I will never lose the sense of myself as a Fat Girl.

I wonder if I ever will. Then again, maybe I never want to.

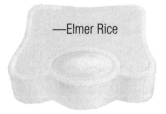

If nature had intended our skeletons to be visible it would have put them on the outside of our bodies.

—Elmer Rice

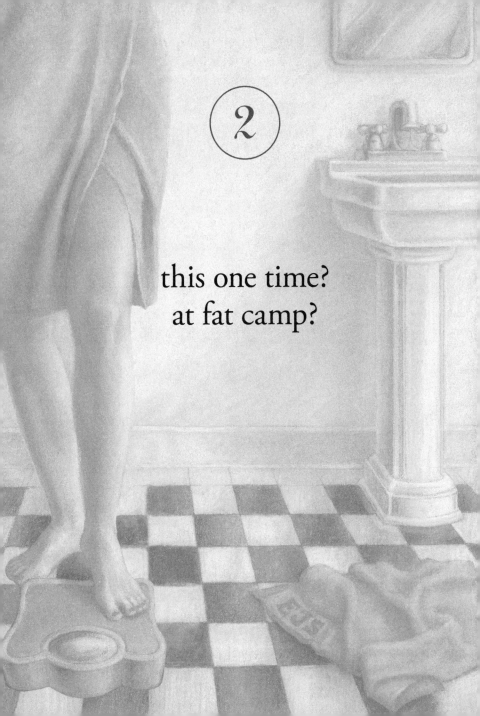

2

this one time?
at fat camp?

Whens and Ifs

By Meegan Foley

I remember sitting on the edge of the dock, my legs dangling in the water. I wore a big New Kids on the Block T-shirt over my swimsuit. I always wore a T-shirt over my bathing suit.

I had gotten my period earlier that year. I tried using tampons but couldn't manage to get them in. I was certain that my hole was convex. I had attached a pad the size of a mattress to my swimsuit. As I sat on the edge of the dock, I willed myself to test the adhesiveness of the pad and slip into the water; but visions of a bloody pad floating by my head when I came up for air kept me seated on the dock, dangling my legs.

I sat in the sun, my father not far from me, scrubbing the bottom of his boat. Both my dad and I liked to clean.

At some point we started to talk about weight. In my younger years I was chubby, then skinny, then chubby, then skinny, then . . . The skinny phases never lasted long. That particular summer was my chubby phase.

"When you lose weight, your confidence will soar and people will respond to you in ways you never imagined," my father said in between dipping his hand into a bucket of bleach and scrubbing the bottom of his boat.

It was always, "When . . . "

Gym Anxiety
By Julie Ridl

Every fat kid has a gym class humiliation story. Or two or three.

I was raised in the strange cocoon that is the U.S. military until the seventh grade. We lived for a while on the shoreline of Subic Bay, Philippines, then a rest stop for the U.S. Navy. A liberty port. Palm trees. Sunsets. Ocean. Warmth. Well, that's not how sailors remember Subic Bay in those days. They remember the place primarily for its nightlife, just off base. But my twelve-year-old eyes saw it as paradise.

I attended military schools, where the curricula varied considerably from the American norm. We had recess, not gym class, when I sat around for an hour or so shooting the breeze with my friends or reading comic books and trashy novels in the shade. I was blissfully unaware of the existence of "physical education." It was too hot to run. We did not hurl balls at one another. We stood around in the heat. Or we climbed trees and sat. I imagined marrying one of the Monkees. I liked Mike. He seemed dangerous. That's how much I knew about danger in those days.

Then we returned to the States, to Sun Prairie, Wisconsin, where I entered civilian life, a civilian school, and the seventh grade in one horrible accident of fate.

Understand: We moved to this little Midwestern cow town directly from the tropics, where our palm-tree-lined yard framed million-dollar sunsets every evening and I slurped the juice of mangoes plucked from my backyard tree. I picked avocados and gardenias in my yard after snorkeling on the most beautiful coral reefs in the world. I had a jungle for my playground. I had free movie theaters, mini-golf, and hobby

37

shops. No kidding. My dad had rank on this base, and by association, so did I. Kids played with me, regardless of my personality or the way I looked. They had no choice.

I was like a kid rock star. Everyone bought my lemonade. I had it all.

But what I didn't know was that I wasn't cool. Not by current U.S. civilian standards. I had lived a beautiful life in the tropics, but returned to the States wearing G.I.-issue horn-rimmed glasses, handmade clothing made to look sort of like what the Sears Catalog was selling.

And then my family and I entered Sun Prairie society to find that no one in the seventh grade wore clothes from the Sears Catalog. Much, much less ersatz Sears Catalog clothes. We were foreigners, spoke with strange accents, dressed in weird clothes and shoes.

And we were military people in a land of civilians. I had been raised to believe that being a Navy family made us a higher order of human being, but it turns out civilian people think just the opposite is true.

So we were odd and out of place, and I was both odd and fat.

An easy target for the cruel wit of seventh graders, I entered my first big school, my first school with many rooms, hallways, staircases, elevators, and lockers. My thick horn-rims slid down my nose, and stuffed in my book bag was my very first gym uniform.

It was a one-piece baby blue jumper with bloomer bottoms. Size Large.

I have been guilty of exaggerating things in the past for the sake of a laugh, but I swear I don't exaggerate this garment. It must have been designed in the 1930s. I've scoured the Net to find an image that comes close to depicting my uniform, but apparently there are parameters of taste on the Internet that prevent posting certain kinds of images.

Bloomer bottoms, snaps up the front, a camp-shirt collar. Crisp cotton/poly blend so it wouldn't wrinkle. Or breathe. The snaps gaped open over my tummy bulge. The elastic dug into my chubby thighs. The one-piece construction meant the thing rode up my bum when I squatted or bent over, for instance, to pick up a dropped ball. And I was nothing if not a ball dropper.

Now, uniforms are meant to equalize the playing field. Right? Put everyone in the same fashion boat? Unfortunately, I lacked the critical piece of information that this school had just dropped their ancient gym bloomers the year of my entry. They'd just adopted cherry red short-shorts and a red-and-white-striped T-shirt.

> Gym anxiety gripped me every other day, wrapping me in icy, clammy skin. I could hear my heart in my ears. I flushed. I panicked. I can still feel the heat of it in my face thirty years later.

I had the only blue bloomers for miles around. And, since my family was on a budget, the uniform just had to do.

It was a bad way to start things at a new school among snotty seventh-grade civilian girls, girls who grew up knowing everyone around them, who had never considered making a new friend, who had never encountered a stranger in their lives—judging by their bubble-gummed, strawberry lip-glossed gapes, which fell open in a perfect wave, girl by girl, as I walked down the halls.

My weirdness left me clinging by my bitten nails to the bottom rung of the social ladder by the middle of the first period of the first day. My complete demotion was pretty well established *before* getting naked with these girls in the locker room and then climbing into my brand-new, last-era, baby blue bloomers. *Before* trying to run around the football field, and coming in dead last. *Before* getting hit in the head with baseballs, in the face with dodge balls, in the gut with basketballs. Accidents, I'm sure. All of them accidents.

I quickly developed all the classic anxiety symptoms before and during gym class that many people have toward math. Gym anxiety gripped me every other day, wrapping me in icy, clammy skin. I could hear my heart in my ears. I flushed. I panicked. Something humiliating happened in every class, leaving me skulking home, taking a different route every day to avoid being reminded of it by classmates. I can still feel the heat of it in my face thirty years later.

I feel it every time I start to run. I feel it every time I walk across the pool, until I can slip into my lane and become invisible again. I feel it in every workout class.

I feel it everywhere except in dance classes. And I know why. During this same time, my mother signed me up for ballet classes taught by a lady at the end of our block. Mrs. Holleman taught ballet in her basement. On the first day, in the first class, wearing my new ballerina tights and my new pink slippers, exactly the right outfit, an outfit that would never change, Mrs. Holleman told me I had beautiful feet. A dancer's feet.

It was a simple thing. And a sweet lie. In dance classes later in life, I learned my feet are not at all good for dance. My toes are all wrong, the arch too high, but this kind little fib gave me a great deal of confidence. I was a chubby, awkward, strange-looking, far-sighted little girl. But I had a dancer's feet, by God.

That just had to mean something.

I worked hard for Mrs. Holleman. Dancing required thought. You must think to dance, remember routines, remember many steps, counts, repeats. In Mrs. Holleman's class, I had potential. In gym class I was a loser who dropped balls and couldn't run around the football field, who came in dead last, with the teacher hovering over her stopwatch, shaking her head, the whole class waiting for me, and then calling out a time that was more than triple that of the faster girls. To peals of laughter. In dance class, I soared. Sort of.

Stopwatches and whistles still grab me by the guts. It takes a lot of work for me to loosen up during a run and remember that I'm working on my own best performance, not racing a bunch of seventh graders. It's three or four sessions in a new yoga class before I remember that everyone there has her mind on her own body, and not on mine.

We're not all runners. Some of us are dancers. Or walkers. We're not all team players. Some of us are loners. But we do all have a way to move that works best for us. None of us were built to sit still. I found mine. I hope you find yours.

And God bless Mrs. Holleman, wherever she is.

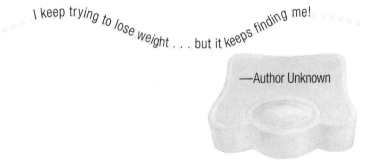

I keep trying to lose weight . . . but it keeps finding me!

—Author Unknown

Eating on Autopilot
By Heather Lockwood

I am about ten years old and my family is sitting down at the dinner table.

I remember the '70s veneer-covered table with its harvest yellow vinyl chairs. I am sitting directly across from my father. His back is toward the cupboards. Mine is to the matching yellow rotary dial phone hanging from the wall. My mother is serving us dinner: goulash, a beef, macaroni, and tomato sauce dish mixed with cheese. My brother is sitting next to me on my left, and my mother is next to him.

Our kitchen table is backed up to the right wall of the kitchen. I'm not sure why—to save space, I suppose. I reach for my glass of milk to wash down my first few bites of dinner and my father shouts out, "I need more milk."

My mother informs him we were out. My father glares at me. "She has more than I do," he barks at my mother without breaking his stare. I look down at my food and continue to eat. I focuse on each bite, hoping the darkening mood will lighten. I take a big gulp of milk to wash down the tasteless food in my mouth. I concentrate on the circle of the glass, the white liquid going down my throat. I am completely off-guard when a big wad of goulash hits my face. "Show off!" says my dad. I am dumbfounded. I was just taking a drink.

But from then on, portions became a big deal. Especially in our family. I learned to eat and drink very, very fast.

I'm eleven going on twelve and my mother informs me I need to go on a diet. She buys me a notebook to track my food. It's velvet with strawberries on the front and I prefer to doodle on the pages instead of logging my calories. I like drawing raccoons with fluffy tails the best. I start my day logging one bowl of Fruit Loops and milk. I finish it quickly, the taste of the cereal barely hitting my lips. I am still hungry and quickly pour another bowl. I eat it fast and omit the second bowl from my log.

My grandfather's living room is the safest in the whole world. He lets me sit in his lap until I'm far too old. I like to share his brown plaid La-Z-Boy recliner, a fancy piece of furniture the likes of which my immediate family has never owned. I am especially fond of the wooden lever on the right that raises and lowers the leg rest with a crisp and distinct metallic noise. My grandfather and I stay up late watching Johnny Carson. He makes batch after batch of popcorn with real butter drizzled over the top. I'm happy. Content. I feel loved. My lack of friends at school no longer plagues my preteen mind. I could care less that I'm already starting to borrow my mother's size 12 clothing. Grandpa sits with me. We eat popcorn. Life is good.

I eat fast. And I eat fair. I count how many pieces of pizza there are when it is delivered. I immediately figure out how much I can have in comparison to my fellow diners. And I wonder about how hungry I will be afterward when the pizza is gone. I barely taste the food. I'm worried about quantity and fill.

Through high school.

Through college.

Through the early part of my marriage.

My obsession with food doesn't seem very apparent. Not to my friends, nor my husband. I would rather die than to admit out loud how I fear three pieces of pizza will not be enough. But the math is always going on inside my head. Will I be full? Will my share be enough?

Where did this obsession come from?

One answer could be that when you are just a little girl eating dinner, you are not prepared for suddenly being punished for having too much. The night my father flung a spoonful of goulash at my face, I wasn't doing anything different than I had any other night of the week. I was drinking my milk just like I was supposed to and suddenly that was wrong. Wrong for having too much. Wrong for showing it off. The moral of that story, "Don't let others see how much you have."

> Starting with my grandfather, I learned how food not only fed my metabolism, but fed my soul as well. I could fill empty spaces with food. I could hide behind food.

Another source of blame could be my mother's poverty during my high school years. There was never much food around the house. Whether or not we'd have enough for dinner was something I thought about often. There was guilt in having too much. So if I did happen to get a little more, I would quickly gulp it down before anyone noticed. On the contrary, I made sure that I always got my fair share. I watched both my mother's and my brother's plates like a hawk.

Then, of course, there is the comfort factor. Starting with my grandfather, I learned how food not only fed my metabolism, but fed my soul as well. I could fill empty spaces with food. I could hide behind food. I could concentrate on taste and let everything else melt away until I sunk into the lethargy that comes from being full.

These days, I manage my compulsion better. I've learned to exercise and eat right. I know what makes up a balanced meal and how much is too much. However, I still go through the math at every meal. I still count the number of Spinach Munchees, an alternative to Totino's Pizza Rolls, in a box and mentally figure there are six for my husband, James, and six for me. God forbid if there is an odd number.

Tonight when I got home from work, I was hungry. I'd eaten smartly all day long. I was ready for dinner, but it was at least an hour away since I still had to cook something. So I grabbed some chips and salsa to settle my hunger. And I devoured chip after chip until I realized a few minutes and a bowl of salsa later, that once again I did not taste my food. I was just filling a space, and filling it fast. I barely had the last bit chewed and swallowed before another chip was entering my mouth. And I thought, *This is it.*

> It doesn't matter if I'm eating organic or vegetarian or high-fiber whole-wheat nuggets of goodness, I'm always going to have to be careful. And mindful of what I'm doing.

This is still where there is work to be done. Because no matter how obsessed with health I become, no matter how full my grocery cart is with organics, no matter how vigorously and religiously I exercise, I will always have this primal desire to just be full. I still have this longing to feel content in my belly and allow that warmth and lethargy to envelop my soul.

It is a hard desire to quell. And it doesn't matter if I'm eating organic or vegetarian or high-fiber whole-wheat nuggets of goodness, I'm always going to have to be careful. And mindful of what I'm doing.

Eating on autopilot is a dangerous thing. It is a habit formed in youth. And it is my constant battle now to overcome that desire for fullness and to break the connection between comfort and food.

The Adventure Begins
By Shauna Marsh

I always thought there would be a great epiphany. I pictured it like the opening credits of *Highway to Heaven*—big fluffy clouds would part, sunbeams would stream down, and perhaps Michael Landon himself would descend. As cherubs plucked at harps he would say unto me, "Now is the time, Shauna. Now you will finally go forth and lose your lard."

But that moment never came. In the end it was all quite anticlimactic. I was slumped in an armchair at my mother's house, back home for Christmas 2000. It was a typical Australian summer afternoon, an energy-sapping 100 degrees. The ceiling fan groaned above me as I slurped away at my second bowl of ice cream. I felt listless and cranky. I hadn't called any of my high school buddies to catch up while we were all home, because I didn't want them to know how big I'd become. I knew I was pretty much settled in for the night, not having the energy to move my 350-pound frame. My only plans for that night consisted of dinner, more dessert, then *It's a Wonderful Life* on the television.

You know, I don't think I feel so wonderful, I thought suddenly. I couldn't remember the last time I felt wonderful.

I looked down at my bulky frame, then looked across to my sister. I pointed to my sprawling stomach and whispered to her, "Right after Christmas, I better do something about this."

And that was that.

Two weeks later on a January evening, the Weight Watchers meeting was packed. It felt like the whole city had made "Lose Weight" their New Year's Resolution. I quickly noticed that I was definitely the heaviest person in the room. It's the first law of fatness: Whenever you enter a room you have to check out the competition and see if there is someone heftier than you are, in case you can squeeze a tiny bit of consolation. No such luck tonight.

> It's the first law of fatness: Whenever you enter a room you have to check out the competition and see if there is someone heftier than you are, in case you can squeeze a tiny bit of consolation.

I also looked at the scale and noticed that it had a 300-pound maximum capacity. I had a sickly feeling I'd be more than that. I'd be one of those people they feature on *A Current Affair* who are so big they have to be taken down to a vehicle-weighing station and queue up with cattle trucks and tourist buses. I was just about to run out the door when my sister suggested we wait until after the meeting to get weighed.

The leader was lovely and motivating. It was then I realized how desperate I felt, how much I wanted her to have the answers.

They were still weighing the New Years Resolutioners after the meeting; there were just so many of us. My sister had only a few pounds to lose, the bitch, but I was so grateful for her presence. She hopped off and smiled, "Your turn."

"Hop on!" said the weigh lady. Her voice was warm.

"I can't," I stammered. I could feel the tears gather again. "I'm too big for the scale."

She looked surprised. I was a heavy girl, but my height tended to disguise the extent of it. "Do you think so?"

"Yes!" My voice was a mere squeak.

She called the leader over and they whispered discreetly. They found an extra weight, another 50 pounds, and hooked it onto the scale to take the capacity up to 360 pounds.

My face burned with shame. I felt so hideous up there. The weigh lady patted my arm. "You look like you're about to crack up! Don't worry. We're here to help you!" she said.

Their kindness made me feel more humiliated and I fought back sobs. Finally they got the scale balanced, and the lecturer looked at me with what I thought was pity, but later I appreciated was genuine compassion. The scale wobbled slightly as I started to cry. I hated myself so much at that moment.

"I'm not going to tell you what the scale read," she said. "I will write it down and we won't worry about goal weights or anything for now. You made the big step coming here tonight. Let's just take it slowly from here."

The leader, the weigh lady, and my sister all looked at me with gentle smiles and sympathy. I just felt sick inside. I know they were being kind, but I didn't feel like being kind to me at that point. I didn't deserve kindness. I was so huge she didn't even want to tell me how much I weighed.

I stepped off the scale and the weight clanged back into the zero position. I knew I was on the verge of sobbing, so I fled into a corner and hid among the Choco-Crisp Bars and POINTS calculators.

The leader came over and hugged me. The warmth of that gesture made my heart crack open, and the enormity of what I had done to my body finally sank in. She told me I'd be okay, that I'd lose the weight and she would help. But all I could think of was how hideous I was, how much I had to lose. I was so overwhelmed I couldn't speak, except to say "sorry" over and over.

I cried in the car all the way home. My sister reminded me that tonight was the toughest step and it would get better from now on. But I had seen my weight written on that card: 352 pounds. I needed to lose more than half of my body to be considered healthy. I was scared, disgusted, and angry. But somehow through that smorgasbord of emotion there was the beginning of a fierce determination. That had been the lowest point of my life, and I knew I didn't want to feel like that anymore.

And that's when the Weblog came into it. I knew I'd need someone to talk to during this monumental journey, but I didn't want to share it with the people in my real life. I wanted to keep the whole process a secret just in case I screwed up. So I started my anonymous journal, "The Amazing Adventures of Dietgirl." Not faster than a speeding bullet, unable to leap tall buildings in a single bound—I hid behind my Lycra-clad roly-poly superhero alter ego and wrote furiously about my weight-loss escapades.

Writing became my calorie-free comfort food. Whenever I wanted chocolate, I distracted my fingers with the keyboard. Writing soothed that overwhelmed feeling. It allowed me to vent, to recognize patterns in my behavior, to keep check of my progress, to sort out old demons in my head.

And then people started to read it. People who were in the same boat and understood how crazy it could be. For someone with very few fat people in her real life, this was a godsend. Finally I could talk about the experience of being fat with people who understood. Kind souls would e-mail words of encouragement, recipes, and exercise tips. Feeling part of a community motivated me even more. I would race home from my weigh-ins to share the results with my online friends.

> Writing became my calorie-free comfort food. Whenever I wanted chocolate, I distracted my fingers with the keyboard.

The hardest thing about diet blogging is not to disappear when you go off the rails. In mid-2002 I went through a rough patch and regained 20 pounds. I stopped writing for three months. I was so ashamed and felt my readers would be disappointed in me.

When I finally returned, I realized I'd been mistaken. They were all understanding and supportive. I realized then what an essential tool Dietgirl had become.

The best part about diet blogging is that the Internet is a very large place. You can be on top of the world after dropping 5 pounds or in the depths of despair because you scarfed down a tub of frosting. But no matter your mood, there is always going to be someone on the Internet who's feeling the exact same way as you and they'll leave a comment or e-mail you to say "I know how you feel."

Knowing you're not alone on the lard-busting journey is more comforting than any bar of chocolate.

According to diet lore, "indulging" or "giving in to temptation" is a "sin." Strangling a few people is a sin. Invading East Timor is a sin. Ethnic cleansing is a sin. Testing nuclear weapons in the Pacific is a sin. I'm sorry, but eating doesn't quite make the grade.

—Kaz Cooke,
Real Gorgeous

To the College and Back
By Erin J. Shea

$\mathcal{M}$y father has taken up running.

I hate that he's done this; I like a chubby daddy. I never understood how my friends with their more streamlined models ever felt safe in their homes with such skinny men ruling the roost. My dad's decision to wake up each morning before sunrise, eat bland, nutritious breakfast bars, and run in circles at the area health club is tantamount to him dropping me off at the bus depot to find lodging elsewhere. For ten years now, he and I have been the heaviest of the four people that make up our family, while my mom and my sister, Kate, are thin as rails.

And now here he goes, off to join the opposing team.

As though the breakfast bars and the oddly flavored sports gum littering our house aren't bad enough, the man has the audacity to start requesting broiled chicken breasts, plain rice, and vegetables for dinner. Even before any of this running business began, he'd subjected my sister and me to a world where Diet Pepsi, skim milk, and water were the only beverages available—but now he is intruding on my territory. Dinner is the only meal where I am guaranteed to consume something breaded, fried, processed, or all of the above. Someone has to put a stop to this nonsense.

"Don't you want a daddy who is skinny?" he said when I asked him why he was doing all of this. "Don't you want a daddy who is in good shape?"

At that age, I wanted a skinny father almost as much as I wanted someone to swoop into our house and steal my collection of Barbie dolls.

But I couldn't tell him that, at least not while he had that glimmer in his green eyes as he explained how much he enjoyed running, how he thought I might like it, too. I didn't want to hurt his feelings and tell him that what I really thought we should do is go to the Weber Dairy for New York Cherry Ice Cream, our favorite.

Despite Dad's preoccupation with All Things Healthy, my report card does not escape his notice. Apparently my good standing in all other subjects won't exempt me from the fascist requirement that all fourth graders understand long division. I steel myself for the inevitable shakedown and the grounding that will follow until I raise my grade in math.

"Erin, do you know you are getting a D in math?"

"But Dad, I . . . " He stops me.

"What do we need to do to get this grade up?" My father has always had this ingenious way of addressing a problem as though it were a group project.

"I have to try harder, Dad."

"Would a tutor help?" I was a smart kid. I would sooner be caught picking my nose and eating what I found during the excavation than have a tutor.

"No. I just need to try harder."

He sighed and looked at the report card and then at me.

"You've been wanting a phone in your room, right?" My desire to have a phone in my room only rivaled my desire to have that phone be a Garfield Phone, as in Garfield the cartoon cat. The receiver doubled as Garfield's back and his eyes would open once you picked it up.

"Yes!"

"I tell you what. You bring that grade up to a B by the end of next semester and I'll get you that Garfield phone for your room—"

"It's a deal," I squealed, interrupting him midsentence.

He finished, "—and. And you have to run with me every morning before school for at least a half a mile."

Oh shit.

The next morning, I was scarfing down a breakfast bar and getting ready for the first of what turned out to be an entire year of predawn runs with Dad. We would make our way down Hunter Avenue, across Jefferson Street, and onto Wilcox, chatting about everything from what we were doing that coming weekend to what I wanted to be when I grew up. By the time we got to Western Avenue, the half-mile point, I would stop and walk while he made his way up the hill to complete the mile. Dad would turn around and continue running until he met up with me and we would take up where we left off in our conversation, walking together the rest of the way home. Sometimes I would get so lost in our conversations, I would run with him for the entire mile. As the months wore on, we would run two miles and come home before my sister and mother were even awake.

By summertime, I was calling all of my friends from the privacy of my room, manually opening and closing Garfield's eyes as we talked about our plans for slumber parties and trips to the pool.

Even better, I had my dad back.

Large, naked raw carrots are acceptable as food only to those who lie in hutches eagerly awaiting Easter.

—Fran Lebowitz

Liar, Liar, Pants Size Higher
By Robyn Anderson

The first time I went on a diet, I was six years old. I don't remember what spurred me into deciding to diet—maybe a round of "Fatty, fatty, two-by-four" from my brothers and their friends, maybe a lifetime of watching my mother diet and exercise, only to stop and gain back what she'd lost, then start the cycle over again. What I do remember is feeling virtuous when I ate only half my sandwich, and how incredibly guilty I felt later that same day, sneaking into the kitchen to steal a cookie.

Sneaking and stealing food was a major theme of my childhood.

I'm the third of four kids, all with a strong sweet tooth. For my entire childhood any kind of sweet treat was put out of our reach. We were allowed a piece of cake or a cookie or two as dessert, but then the container was put away and we weren't allowed more, and probably with good reason since the four of us would surely have consumed everything in no time flat. I remember one of my brothers getting caught stealing brownies. He got in big trouble, and years later I got punished for stealing chocolate chip cookies from my parents' closet.

My mother and sister sat in the living room, and I stood in the doorway to be sure they were involved in whatever they were watching, then walked quietly down the hall and into my parents' room. I opened the plastic container, took just one cookie, stuffed it into my mouth and swallowed on the way back down the hallway, my heart pounding and cheeks flushed with the illicit thrill of eating something I wasn't supposed to have. After four or five such trips, my mother got suspicious and followed me back down the hall where she caught me with my hand—literally—in the cookie jar.

A few years later, desperate for the taste of something sweet, I snuck into the kitchen, grabbed a tub of Swiss Miss hot chocolate mix and a spoon, and then went back to my room, where I ate right from the container. A moment later my father walked in without knocking. I desperately tried to hide the mix under the pillow sitting in my lap, but the chocolate powder around my mouth gave me away. After a brief struggle, he walked out of the room carrying the tub of mix. A few minutes later, after washing my face, I followed him out to the living room where I tried to strike up a conversation, an attempt cut short when he said, "Don't talk to me."

I ate in secret for a good part of my life, eating normally around other people, and then again when I was alone, stuffing food into my mouth as quickly as possible, barely tasting it, then covering the smell with gum or breath mints.

I was fourteen the first time I went to NutriSystem. It was brand new at the time, a diet mostly made up of prepackaged foods, and my mother and I were suckered in by the ads and the revolutionary idea: prepackaged foods and no decisions to make, ever! We visited the office and in no time we left with a bag of prepackaged food and sheets of instructions. For the first week, I followed the diet to the letter, eating everything I was supposed to, and no more. The day of my first weigh-in, my mother was out of the house running errands, and I was home alone. I had eaten my breakfast, but I was starving. Since no one else was around, I searched frantically for something to eat. In the freezer I found a shake. My brother worked at an ice cream store and would bring home the occasional dish of ice cream or shake made of odd flavors. I grabbed a spoon and scooped some of the shake out of the cup. It was made with bubble gum ice cream, and as nasty as that was, I still ate half of what was there before putting it back in the freezer, shaking with guilt and worry over what my weigh-in would reveal. I skipped lunch and was rewarded by a 7-pound loss that evening.

I don't know how it all started, but I do know that by the time I'd been attending NutriSystem for six months I had developed my own system. Weigh-in was on Tuesday afternoon. From Tuesday night to Friday, I'd eat everything I could get my hands on, always in secret. I'd stock up on food in advance, biking down to the corner store to buy doughnuts and cakes and hiding them in my room in places where my mother wouldn't find them. From Friday to Tuesday, I ate as little as I could possibly get away with, telling my mother I had already eaten or would eat later. As time passed and I stopped losing weight, I stopped eating on Thursday instead of Friday. I'd go to weigh-in and I'd have lost a tiny amount of weight or nothing or even gained some, and I'd go back out to where my mother was sitting in the waiting room and lie to her about how much I'd lost.

For Christmas that year, I got the book *Starving for Attention*, an autobiography chronicling Cherry Boone O'Neill's struggles with anorexia and bulimia. To me, it was almost a how-to manual. Thus began my flirtation with bulimia. I tried seriously to make myself throw up after a binge, but I had a pretty cast-iron stomach and could never force myself. I started shoplifting laxatives from a store downtown, stuffing them in my purse just out of sight of the security mirrors. At first, after a binge I'd take six or seven laxatives, but I quickly worked my way up to an entire package at a time.

Here's a quick and nasty fact of life: When you're taking an *entire* package of laxatives at a time, even if you take them in the afternoon when you're at home and near a bathroom, at some point you're going to lose control of your bowels when you are nowhere near a bathroom. I began wearing maxi pads as diapers to protect my jeans (and by the time the school day started, there was very little in my system to pass through my bowels, so the maxi pads were enough protection). I wanted to stop taking the laxatives, but the days of being able to eat nothing, of being able to lie in bed and feel my stomach growling, feeling as if I were eating myself from the inside out and loving the feeling, were gone. I could no longer starve myself from Thursday to Tuesday, as much as I wanted to, as much I swore to myself that I would. So I had to take the laxatives to get the food I was eating in private in my room out of my system, and then I had to get up ten times in the night to go to the bathroom after they kicked in.

To this day, I can't swallow a small, coated pill without gagging.

Eventually, even with the laxatives, I stopped losing weight and sometimes gained. Once, I stepped on the scale to find that I'd gained 4 pounds in one week. I tried to put it off to having my period, but the nurse looked at my hands and ankles and said that if it were water retention there'd definitely be some bloat in one place or the other. She began lecturing me about sticking exactly to the foods I was supposed to eat and to getting some exercise, and I sat there and meekly nodded. She reminded me of how much money my parents had spent to help me lose weight, and I sat and listened, but I hated her, thinking, *How can you be so stupid? You're a nurse. How can you not see this?*

I went out to the waiting room and told my mother I'd lost a pound and a half. My mother was thrilled and I stood there as she gushed to the receptionist about how well I was doing. The nurse who'd weighed and lectured me came out in time to hear my mother say again, "A pound and a half this week, that's good!" She gave me a look and asked my mother if she could speak to her alone. My mother sent me out to the car to wait, and when she came out she was furious. At one point she said, "It's not that you gained weight; it's that you lied!"

But I was sure that was a lie, and that all she cared about was that I had gained.

A few weeks later my father picked me up from ballet practice. I had ballet practice on Thursday evenings, and after practice let out I'd walk from the ballet studio to the library. But before I went to the library, I'd make a side trip to the store, where I'd study the candy bars for a long, long time before choosing two or three of them to buy. I'd go to the library and sit at a table, stuffing a candy bar in my mouth as unobtrusively as possible while looking through a pile of books I'd pulled off the shelf.

On the night in question, my father picked me up and then told me to wait in the car while he ran into the store. I sat in the backseat and decided that I could get away with eating another candy bar while I waited. When my father got back in the car, he sat there for a second and then said, "Do you think I can't smell the chocolate?" He refused to talk to me on the way home. When we got home, I went straight to my room, but I could hear him out in the living room telling my mother. I heard my sister's voice telling my mother that she'd seen a box of doughnuts under my bed earlier that day, and then my mother came into my room, slamming the door open. She looked under my bed and said, "What the fuck is *this*?"

She picked up two boxes of laxatives and held them out to me. I couldn't look at her. She took the laxatives, the doughnuts, and my duffel bag, and she left the room, slamming the door behind her. A few minutes later I was still staring at the floor when she came back in.

"Where did you get these?" she asked, and I told her, though I didn't tell her that I'd shoplifted them. "Don't you think they *knew* what you were going to do with them?"

Of course, she had no idea that I'd been taking laxatives for more than a month and she had no way of knowing I'd been shoplifting them, either. I said nothing, still staring at the floor. She lectured me for several minutes, and I said nothing.

Finally, sounding resigned, she said, "Do you want to stop going to NutriSystem?" and I said, "Yes." She said, "All you had to do was *say* that you wanted to stop going. Why didn't you just say so?" I thought, *Because when I gained weight, you reminded me of how much money you'd already spent. Because my weight is the most important thing about me and the only thing you care about.*

But I said nothing.

I never went back to NutriSystem, although my mother did try to talk me into going back. A counselor from Nutri-System called later to cajole me into going back, but for once in my life I held fast. It took some time, but I gained back every pound I'd lost and more.

I'd like to say that I never walked across the threshold of another diet program, but I tried NutriSystem not once, not twice, but three times more. The funny thing with fat woman is that often we think back to the times we successfully lost weight and think not that the program failed us, but that we failed the program and should give it another honest try. The last time I tried NutriSystem, I lost 50 pounds before I gave up and stopped going. I half-heartedly tried Weight Watchers once or twice, but never lost any significant amount of weight while attending. I tried diets at home at various points in my life—Atkins, Cabbage Soup Diet, just plain starving myself, once for an entire week at a time, eating nothing and drinking only water and soda—but nothing worked in the long run.

59

I was fifteen when I stopped going to NutriSystem that first time. I weighed around 150 pounds, and as soon as I stopped attending Nutri-System, I started gaining weight. When I was thirty-two, I stepped on the scale and found that I'd eaten my way up to a high of 362 pounds.

I'd love to say that stepping on the scale and seeing that number, hearing it echo in my brain, three *hundred* and sixty-*two* was enough to make me immediately start working out and eating right, but that's not the way it happened. It wasn't one big moment but several little ones that got me going.

First of all, my husband, who weighed only a little more than I, who had matched me bite for bite through our entire relationship, had started to lose weight. When you're used to someone else eating the way you eat and moving as little as you do and they suddenly change the status quo, that can be a scary thing. It shakes up your world. I couldn't count on him sitting with me in front of the TV and stuffing junk food in his face anymore. We started listening to a set of Tony Robbins tapes and I joke that I started to exercise so that Fred wouldn't make me listen to the ass-numbing boredom of those tapes (sorry, Tony) anymore.

Around the time that was happening, I went to Wal*Mart. As I drove along the front of the store looking for a parking space as close to the building as possible, I saw an elderly woman walk out of the store. She was extremely overweight and moved slowly, struggling for every step, and I felt a little frisson of fear go down my spine. I thought, *What the hell am I doing? I'm throwing it all away. I can move easily now, but in*

I'd love to say that stepping on the scale and seeing that number, hearing it echo in my brain, three *hundred* and sixty-*two,* was enough to make me immediately start working out and eating right, but that's not the way it happened.

thirty years, that's going to be me, if I can even walk by then. If I'm even alive *in thirty years.*

It took a few days after that, but one morning I woke up and stared at the ceiling, and I knew with a sense of finality that I had *no choice*. If I kept eating and not moving, I *would* be that woman. I was in pretty good shape for a Fat Chick, but there was no way that could continue. I had *no choice*.

So I began exercising with my husband, which at the beginning was running in place in the pool in our backyard for ten minutes every night. I graduated to doing walking tapes inside—which kicked my ass for a long time—and eventually started walking outside. I'm never going to be a person who loves to exercise or craves exercise every day (I shudder at the thought), but I keep that thought in the back of my mind, and although there are times when I can't force my butt out of bed for love or money, a lot of times I think, *I have no choice*—and that's enough to get me moving.

Stressed spelled backward is *desserts.* Coincidence? I think not!
—Author Unknown

Enjoy Your Milkshake
By Lori Ford

There was this diner across the street from my pediatrician's office that my mom would take me to after every doctor's appointment. After a visit to the doctor's office that included needles, I would always order a chocolate milkshake and spin around on the barstool. Those milkshakes have always been the best I've ever had. Maybe because I'd spend the most horrifying moments of my life looking forward to them or it was just the way they'd relax me. Calm me. Bring me back to my safe world.

At six, my doctor consulted the all-knowing height/weight charts and declared that I wasn't overweight but I was "headed in that direction." He gave my mother a strict diet meal plan for me to follow. The chocolate milkshake after this visit would take on a whole new meaning, one that I would become all too familiar with during the rest of my life: the last day before beginning a diet. The milkshake suddenly seemed tastier, creamier, and more divine. Right then, in that moment, that milkshake had become a forbidden food, making its allure all the more powerful.

> Enjoy your milkshake, because tomorrow you start your diet.

Enjoy your milkshake, because tomorrow you start your diet.

I think it was most difficult for me during breakfast. I'd always try to wake up early on Saturday mornings to watch a marathon of cartoons. I was usually up before anyone else, and I'd make my own bowl of Lucky Charms for breakfast. But on my diet I had to endure hunger pains until my mother would wake and cook me one scrambled egg, one piece of bacon, and one slice of dry toast. The only thing I remember about my first diet was the breakfast.

I had a birthday party to attend in my neighborhood, and my mother, following sound diet advice, had me eat before going to the party so I wouldn't be hungry. She made me promise not to eat anything at the party because it would break my diet. Once at the party the birthday girl's mother wouldn't hear of me not having cake and ice cream, so I had some; then I went ahead and had some chips as well.

When I got home, my mother asked me if I had anything to eat and I told her what I had eaten. She was very angry with me and told me I had to go ride my bike around the block ten times, immediately. I cried the whole way. It was the first time exercise became punishment.

At around age eight, I had my first binge episode. I ate an entire bag of Doritos and involuntarily threw them up. I didn't think much about it at the time, except that I should never eat Doritos again. I don't remember why I ate the entire bag. Was it emotional, related to my parents' divorce that was occurring around that time?

> My mother told me I had to go ride my bike around the block ten times, immediately. I cried the whole way. It was the first time exercise became punishment.

During my prepubescent years my mother, hawklike, watched what I ate in her presence. When I was out of her line of sight, I would sneak whatever I could. I remember one summer sailing trip when my mother turned to me and told me my face was very puffy and I must have gained weight. I couldn't be off my diet for a weekend without it being noticeable in my face.

Summer vacations were spent flying to Florida to visit my grandparents. My mother would ask my grandmother not to let me go off my diet, but my grandmother, who also had a weight problem, would throw out my diet and let me eat whatever I wanted. There, I ate to excess as if I were making up for lost time. My mother would be noticeably upset to see me when I got home and would promptly put me back on a diet.

After puberty it was me who insisted on putting myself on impossible diets, usually starvation diets. I would buy Dexatrim and take more than recommended, thinking it would work twice as fast. I would sit in class completely distracted by this weird head-tingling sensation, a side effect of too many of the appetite suppressants. I would take NoDoze during the day thinking the extra energy would increase my metabolism. It would make me paranoid and jumpy, though I got a lot of ironing done. Exercise was never for fun once I was in high school. It was only to lose weight, and I'd avoid it whenever possible, choosing to starve over exercise.

There was a point where I wanted to be bulimic. The idea that I could eat all I wanted and not ingest the calories was magical to me. I'd kneel over the toilet with my finger in my throat and try unsuccessfully to make myself throw up. I'd be so frustrated that I couldn't do this one thing, this one thing that could solve all my problems. I once got the idea to eat Pop-Tarts over the sink and chew them but spit them out instead of swallowing. I tried it a few times but never really satiated the need to eat the Pop-Tart. There was something lost in spitting out liquid chunks of chocolate Pop-Tarts.

I continued the crash diets. The weight would come off quickly and I'd put it back on just as fast. My friends would often make fun of me for bringing yogurt to school for lunch and I'd often cheat and eat at fast-food restaurants, dieting around what my friends could see. My weight was constantly up and down. It was difficult to tell exactly how much because in the 1980s, the style was to wear everything baggy.

I always felt fat and insecure about my size no matter what size I was. If a boy didn't like me, I was sure it was because of my weight. If I was overweight I never dated, and when I was thin I was a complete wreck about my size and wondered if guys would like me.

Even when thin, I was a Fat Girl in a thin girl's body.

Nestle Crunch, Burger King, and Camryn Manheim

By Monique van den Berg

Nobody ever taught me to love my body. As much as I loved to bike ride and swim and play outside when I was a kid, as active as I could potentially have been even with my "baby fat," the nightmarish world of elementary school stamped it all out of me: one irresponsible phys ed coach in particular.

My coach had no tolerance for me. I ran laps the slowest, had less stamina than the rest of the kids. My teachers seemed to love me—I connected this with the fact that I was smart. My coach seemed to hate me—I connected this with the fact that I was hopeless at sports. I remember this coach encouraging the athletic kids to pick the best people for their teams by pointing out who should be left on the bench: me.

I retreated to what I was good at, academic work. And as I became more and more self-conscious, more isolated and bookish, more friendless and insecure, I grew to hate and dread physical activity. It wasn't fun anymore.

I was even awkward enough to break my bones doing things like jumping rope and playing dodge ball. I grew fearful of pain and injury. I just want to reach out and hug that little girl. I wish my parents had seen it happening to me and had known what to do to stop it.

I always used to blame my mother for passing on her issues. She has been significantly overweight—even obese—for my entire life. She answered all of my teenage emotional fluctuations by inviting me to raid the cookie jar or by baking me a cake. Then every so often she'd feed me nothing but string beans, pickled beets, and nonfat ice cream for a week.

Food was punishment for being fat, and food was reward.

All my childhood memories involve food. I remember being three years old and having my hand slapped by an uncle because I was reaching for a doughnut. I remember sneaking out of my bed, age nine, to eat stale cookies. I remember being told when I was twelve that my eyes were bigger than my stomach. For me, food was always a guilty, forbidden thing. It was a series of tests that I could never successfully pass.

I vividly remember the day my mother pointed at the numbers on the scale as they bounced between 99 and 100 and said, "That's okay, just don't get any bigger. I don't want you to be like me." And then she cried. I was fourteen. I grew to be 5'10", all the while convinced that I was fat if I weighed more than 100 pounds.

> All my childhood memories involve food. I remember being three years old and having my hand slapped by an uncle because I was reaching for a doughnut.

And as a result, there has never been a time that I was not negotiating a relationship with food—my best friend and my worst enemy and, in some particularly complicated way, my parent (sustenance, love, approval, reprimand . . .).

When I was a teenager, my parents started a vending-machine business. I got to be very good at sneaking into the inventory—my favorite things were the granola bars, the brownies, the gingersnaps, and the Nestle Crunch bars. I think my mother always knew what I was doing, what I was eating the moment her back was turned. She acknowledged it because she did it, too. I was a food hoarder, a secret binge eater.

I didn't have any friends for many years. Books were my friends. So was food.

When I was in elementary school, we used to get Burger King delivered to our classroom on Wednesdays. That delicious-smelling pile of burgers tormented me. I used to have fantasies of an entire truckful of Burger King hamburgers pulling up in front of my school, and I would get in the truck, roll around in the hamburgers, and eat as many as I wanted.

That's why college, for me, was all about the freedom of the Burger King drive-through. And the late-night pizza that we could order with our student meal cards. And the chocolate cake that nobody would have to know I was eating, in my dorm room, alone. Needless to say, that's why college was where I put on most of my excess weight.

I thought about food a lot. I think about food a lot, to this day. A great meal does make me happy. Anticipating a treat lifts my spirits. And I can relive the top five meals I've ever had, in exquisite detail. When I've had a bad day, I try to make it all better with Oreo cookies or a club sandwich, extra bacon.

And that's why I put on another 50 pounds or so in my twenties. I had a job I hated and was in a bad relationship, and some days the only thing that got me through it was the knowledge that I could have Chinese food for dinner. My unhappiness manifested itself as fat. I had a boss who was a horror-movie caricature of a competitive female executive. She harped on all of the women who worked there. Our clothes were ugly, our haircuts were awful, and we were fat. I don't mean that she would restrict herself to subtle comments, either. She bought one woman a gym membership. She sent someone else to her beauty parlor—and her therapist. She gave us money to buy clothes.

One day, she told me that I should be able to "dress like that fat lawyer on *The Practice*. She always looks professional, at least." I didn't have Camryn Manheim's wardrobe budget, but I tried anyway, wearing pantyhose and blazers to a job where I never met a single client. And then I went home every night and ate a gallon of ice cream because "dress like that fat lawyer"? Screw you, lady—on Camryn's behalf *and* mine.

My unhappiness manifested itself as fat. And then I changed my life—my job, my relationship, my living situation—and the pounds dropped away. At least the unhappiness pounds did. But I still had the "food is comfort and love" pounds. Then I took up bike riding, which helped. Then I joined Weight Watchers, which helped more. Then I started on the long, lifetime process of renegotiating my relationship with food.

Somewhere along the way, I decided to start a Weblog to chronicle my weight loss. The goal was public accountability, a way to examine my own patterns, to get support and advice, and to become a part of a community of smart, intelligent writers. These writers who believed, as I did, that being overweight was not the worst sin in the world, and that there was a way to be healthy and happy and at ease with eating that had nothing to do with one's pants size.

It wasn't the women at the Weight Watchers meetings that I wanted to emulate—those scary women so obsessed that they were talking about ways to say "no" to a piece of wedding cake *at their own weddings*. It was the women I met online who I truly admired. These women who understood that it was okay to love food and not go to war with it. They understood the siren call of warm chocolate chip cookies. And most of all, they understood that none of us—not me, not them, and not Camryn Manheim, either—had to hate our body in order to change it for the better.

> To eat is a necessity, but to eat intelligently is an art.
> —La Rochefoucauld

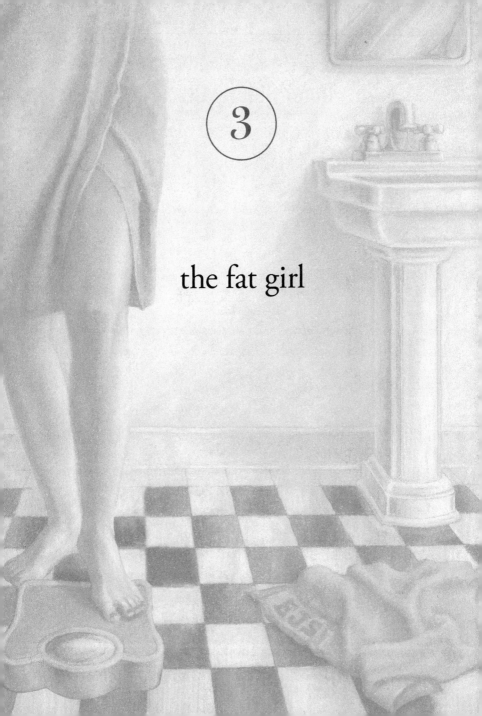

3

the fat girl

Inner Skinny Chick

I don't have an inner Fat Girl. I have an inner Skinny Chick instead. She's just as much of a saboteur, an irritant, even a heartbreaker. Trust me on this.

I was a skinny child. The pounds didn't show up until college, that infamous "freshman 5," which was really 10, or was it 15? Back then, all I had to do to lose weight was think, *Oh, I should lose weight,* and a week or two later I'd fit into my leotards and leather pants again.

That's wonderful, that's what you want, right? Pleasure and pride in your body as well as your mind. But what happens when you gain weight later on? Let's say you've had a stressful year at a job demanding fifteen-hour days and lots of "Yes, sir, right away, sir" obsequiousness that doesn't come naturally to you? You eat the doughnuts always on hand and you unbutton your pants every time you sit down. Then you buy a larger size.

And what happens when you decide to take that weight off? You look in the mirror and you only see the jowls and the saddlebags of fatty deposits and the ripple of too many cells bulging under your skin. Time to do something about it. But what? The inner Skinny Chick whispers in your ear, "That'll be off in a week, you'll see." And you believe her.

By Tamar Bihari

A week goes by. You work at it harder than you ever have. Two weeks go by. The number on the scale goes down. The pants feel maybe a little looser. You walk into the bedroom after your shower and get a glimpse of your naked body in the mirror. You look like someone else's hand-me-down clothes. You're frustrated and angry. This isn't supposed to happen! It's supposed to be easy, not hard! The pounds are supposed to melt off; they're supposed to flee screaming for mercy.

What do you do when you're frustrated and angry? When you hate yourself? You eat. And while you stand there in the kitchen, grabbing handfuls of tortilla chips and stuffing them into your mouth—too many at once—you forget your uncomfortable body. You're still skinny, you see. Your inner Skinny Chick has told you so.

The only way to win against a skinny bitch like this is to tell her—tell yourself—the truth. To shed your clothes and stand in front of the mirror with all the lights on. To take a good look at the flab on your inner thigh, the roundness of your cheeks, the slope of your abdomen. To admit this is you. And it's not going to go away in a day or a week or even a month. This is you and you're not skinny anymore but that's okay; there's freedom in that. Freedom to change yourself. Not overnight—the time for that is long gone. This change happens over time, months or even years. And it starts with owning your body. Right now.

My Skinny Chick is quiet these days. And I'm taking the pounds off. My way.

Doormats Grow Fat
By Julie Ridl

I had breakfast the other day with a friend who manages the Human Resources department for a giant company. She's grown good at understanding basic differences among people. We were marveling at another friend's ability to carve out a very defined way of working at one important project at a time, his success at avoiding picking up other projects that really need to be done to focus on his priority projects.

I said, "I want that to be my next job, a job where I get to focus on one project at a time."

She just *looked* at me.

"Do you think you *could*?"

"I'd love it," I lied. And then, later, I had to admit, there is no way I'd be able to work that way.

That is, I haven't yet mastered the art of saying no. I haven't learned to limit what I take on. If there is a need or a project in my way that someone else has dropped, and I find myself tripping over it, I'm likely to pick it up, along with everything else on my plate, and try to do that, too.

Because I'm a doormat.

I am not made into a doormat by virtue of being a girl, by virtue of my ability, my experience, my doggedness, my attention to detail, by any virtue at all. I have been a doormat because I need to please people. Or maybe because I fear displeasing them.

Oddly enough, it has been weight loss that has helped me identify my self-imposed doormattedness. By risking disappointing people when I choose to work out, choose to cook different foods or choose not to cook at all, choose to spend time learning about nutrition, finding sources for less processed foods, I learned that I wasn't risking anything at all.

No one cares what I don't do. It's what I *do* that they focus on. And by taking on too much, always, the people in my life see me as an over-committed, unavailable, distraught, and distracted person. If I chose to do less, in fact, I would likely come off as more sane, more focused, and oddly enough, more accomplished. More complete as a person. More available and thus more loving and lovable. Seriously.

I would love to figure out how to study the relationship between doormattiness and heaviness. I hypothesize a pretty interesting correlation there.

My hypothesis: Doormats grow fat. With no time to exercise, no time to prepare healthy meals, doormats fly from duty to duty, grabbing candy bars and soda between commitments, believing they have no time to chew their food or prepare a fresh vegetable.

I *would* conduct this study, but frankly, I'm not taking on any new assignments at the moment.

See what I did there? That's a start. That's called "learning to say no," and it's a very sane way to live. If you've never done it before, the next two weeks are a good time to try it out. Here are some phrases I've been trying out:

- I'm not taking on any new assignments right now.
- My plate is full, sorry.
- My cup runneth over at the moment.
- Can I get back to you in 2010?
- This resource is endangered.
- I can't this year.
- My quarter's overbooked.
- I'm stretched too far as it is, sorry.

- I wish I could do all I'd like to do, but I can't.
- It's a worthy cause all right, but there are so many, and I'm booked.
- Sorry, but I needed to reprioritize all of my commitments, and this one didn't make my list this year.
- Sorry, but more pressing personal matters are taking my time right now.
- I'm so sure!

And my personal favorite:
- No.

People who say yes become targets for people who say no. Try not to make things worse for other doormats when you're saying no. Don't direct people their way. Just say no, and leave it there. And, you know you really don't need to explain "busy." We all understand what busy is.

When you say no, you protect yourself and your time. You say you are one human with a finite amount of time in your day, in your week, in one lifetime. You preserve peace and quiet, and time to do things you actually enjoy, things that feed your heart and mind. With a reasonable number of items on our to-do lists, we can make time to prepare and sit down to eat our meals; we restore our dignity and humanity.

No more anxious eating to fuel fruitless living. Say no.

Self-delusion is pulling in your stomach when you step on the scales.
—Paul Sweeney

A Better Girl
By Heather Lockwood

$\mathcal{E}$ ach weekday morning when the alarm goes off at 5:15 A.M., I have an internal struggle. As I listen to the inflectionless voices on Public Radio inform me of the political instability of the Middle East or how a new gene that controls obesity has been discovered in rats, I roll around and consider staying in bed another hour. I stretch and scratch my dog's belly and then rationalize why my body needs an extra hour of sleep. I tell myself that I really don't need to get up because I worked out yesterday. Or I promise myself I'll work out in the afternoon if I can just snooze another forty-five minutes. Of course, this argument usually gets quashed as I wake up and realize that working out at any other time of the day will probably not be an option. I'll hate myself if I don't get up. My day won't go well if I don't start it right and starting it right, for me, means exercise. With that, I pull my body out of bed at almost 5:30 A.M. on the dot and head to the bathroom where I brush my teeth, put on my workout gear, pee, and wash my face. Although, I don't always do those things in that precise order. Sometimes peeing can't wait.

I like this time of the day, when I get up to enjoy it. The dogs are still slow to rise so I don't have to worry about them getting underfoot. The house is quiet. And as I stand in the kitchen packing my office food for the day (salad to go with my Lean Cuisine for lunch, fruit for a midday snack), I look out the window at the dark house next door. I feel slightly superior when I gaze at the unlit windows. I know my neighbors are probably still in bed, yet here I am. I'm up at 5:30 A.M. because working out, for me, is that important.

I leave the house twenty minutes later, pack the car, and arrive at my health club by 6 A.M. Nancy at the front desk always greets me by name. Her freckled face is always awake and inviting even in my grumpiest of states. At the gym, I vary my routine. Some mornings I take a spinning class. Others I spend working out with weights. If it is summer, I can be found in the pool training for one of my upcoming triathlons because swimming is by far my weakest sport.

There are other mornings when I don't drive to the club. I stay home instead and run around the neighborhood. We live a mile from a small lake. The distance around it is exactly 3.25 miles. Running to the lake, around it, and back is about 5 miles. I like these mornings when I'm out and the sun is rising. It is a special day when I'm lucky enough to spot a crane or baby geese on my jog. I return home where I stretch out on my deck and do some abdominal work before heading inside to make coffee and shower for work.

Mornings spent at the gym are a little different. I shower there and get ready with many of the ladies I've gotten to know over the years. We smugly call ourselves regulars. I'm especially fond of the generous ones who will share an outlet or hair dryer when needed. We silently glare at the selfish regulars. The ones who hold spots at the countertop by spreading their makeup and brushes out before they even need to use the space.

When I leave the gym to drive to work, I usually stop at the coffee shop just down the street. I order a 20-ounce dark roast, no room for cream, that I take with me on the commute. And as I drive through traffic to start my day, I am calm and peaceful even when the interstate is crowded and backed up. Sometimes I even find myself smiling at my fellow drivers, although it is rare that I get a similar expression in return.

Once I'm at work, it is a whole different ball game. Immediately, I get sucked into whatever issues happen to be going on at the moment.

But I'd like to say that I handle everything better after my morning ritual. My mornings are almost Zenlike and allow me to enter each day with a fresh perspective and a calm demeanor.

I can't say that has always been the case.

On the flip side, in prior years I'd enter my workday with the same grumpiness I shared with the rest of the world. I had a 30-pound overweight chip on my shoulder and life just seemed harder. Getting up was always a struggle. I was constantly tired and irritable. When the alarm would go off in the morning, the Fat Girl that I was would hit the snooze over and over until she knew that she could no longer put off starting another day.

She would crawl into the shower and curse the size of her belly as she washed her hair and scrubbed her body. She would grab onto the fat rolls in the middle and imagine cutting them off with a knife. Just take off the fat, she would muse, take off the fat. If only it worked that way. . . .

When she would get out of the shower, she would immediately put on her clothing. Staring into bathroom mirrors naked was not one of her favorite pastimes. And once the drying off and combing of hair were done, she'd head straight for the kitchen where she'd eat one, make that two bowls of sugary cereal. Lucky Charms were her favorite although Crackling Oat Bran was a good one, too. Her coffee always contained cream and sugar and while she gulped down her breakfast, life didn't seem so bad. Of course, she would return to the bathroom shortly thereafter and the calming effects of the food would already be wearing off. She needed to do her hair, so she would be faced with herself in the mirror once again. She hated her reflection. She hated the puffiness in her face. She worked extra hard on her hair to give it just the right volume. She felt that the more volume to the style, the more flattering to the face. So, she teased and sprayed. She applied makeup with the heavy-handedness of a pro. She always wore the hole enchilada: concealer, foundation, blush, eye shadow, mascara, and lip-gloss. Like the hair, her approach was "more is better." More was more concealing. And when you live with 30-plus extra pounds, you need all the concealing you can get.

Getting dressed was always the most dreaded part of getting ready in the mornings. Sometimes she'd delay the activity by taking another stop into the kitchen for a piece of toast, maybe two. Eventually, she'd have to face her closet, the closet that was chock-full of clothing yet contained nothing to wear. Too small, too tight, too hot, too light, too out of date, too revealing. Everything was too, too, too. There were probably only four or five things in there she even liked to wear, four or five things she felt didn't make her look fat or old or frumpy. Those four or five things were always black and baggy and usually came from Target or Old Navy, stores that allowed her to shop for plus sizes without big "plus size" signs overhead.

Eventually, she'd settle on something. Then she would examine it in the mirror from every angle and vantage point. She would examine her profile and her rear. She'd cross her hands in front of her, then put them on her hips. She'd stare at herself in the mirror, and then glare at the double chin this created. She'd smooth out wrinkles in the front of her shirt and then hold in her stomach. And at some point she'd give up, sigh at the mirror, and head for the door.

Yet, even though she had escaped her mirror, the vision of herself would stay in her mind. She would go over her posterior and anterior and wonder why she looked so fat. She would jealously fixate on her younger coworker at the office, the one who looked good in everything she wore yet never seemed to put too much care into the process. At this thought, the Fat Girl would become more aggressive as she drove her way into work. These thoughts were needle pricks in her mind that only fed her aggression, which she took out on slow drivers and uncooperative stoplights. By the time she arrived at work, she was already sick of the world.

And that is how I greeted the day, every day. It makes me both sad for then and thankful for now.

My Fat Girl wasn't pathetic, however. Let's make that clear right now. She was funny and colorful. She always had the office in stitches, telling jokes all day long. And she was best at being critical of everything and everybody. She probably spent so much time mentally critical of herself that doing it to others was a release.

My Fat Girl had a sense of style, too. Despite the fact that getting dressed was a chore, she'd spend hour after hour with *In Style* magazine and *Glamour*. She knew what was a "do" and a "don't" and she never ceased to share this vast knowledge with her friends and family. She knew what hair products all the celebrities used and she invested large amounts of money in a collection that amassed underneath her bathroom sink. Each purchase was another chance at hope. Another opportunity to fix that reflection in the mirror and deflect from the real issue that was just too hard to face.

I'd like to add that my Fat Girl was also lucky. She had an amazing husband and family who made her feel like a million bucks no matter what she was wearing or how she looked. She had a hard time believing their compliments when contrasted with the inner critic, but she was thankful they were not so harsh.

My Fat Girl spent a lot of time celebrating. She celebrated everything and with lots of food. She baked cakes and cookies for her coworkers; she fixed feasts for herself and her husband. Every activity had a food associated with it. Movies meant popcorn. Football meant Buffalo wings. Basketball was margaritas and unlimited chips and salsa. She was a culinary artist. Her coworkers went bonkers for her chocolate-covered potato chips and fudgy brownies that contained more than a stick of butter.

She always had candy, too. She loved to share and would stock the office candy dish with Hershey Miniatures and Dove Promises. She would damn the Reese's Peanut Butter Cups as she snacked on them midday but then returned for more. She'd then tempt her coworkers so that they, too, would take part in the activity of passing the workday in a flurry of chocolate and sugar.

My Fat Girl called herself a foodie. She would proudly declare her love for all things carbohydrate and make no apologies for her love affair with food. Yet when she would return home in the evening, she would curse the cravings she felt she could not control. She figured exercise was pointless. Besides, it was a lot of work.

So she would vegetate on the couch in an effort to escape the reality of her body and her life. She loved TV. She had a show for every night of the week. Thursdays were her favorite, so she usually paired the viewing with pizza and beer. And as she filled her stomach and her mind, she would forget the woman she hated. She would ignore the inner critic. She would retreat into the cushions on the couch. It was there that she felt safe and at home.

> My Fat Girl called herself a foodie. She would proudly declare her love for all things carbohydrate and make no apologies for her love affair with food.

Of course, years later, it is rare that I spend an evening on the couch eating and watching TV—even on the weeknights, as hard as that is to believe. On the odd occasion that I do, I am usually regretful of my inactivity. I hate to waste time, perhaps because I wasted so much of it as a Fat Girl. I wasted time on the couch, time in front of the mirror, and time just seething with jealousy over what friends and celebrities had. There was so much time wasted that I will never get back.

I can't pinpoint what exactly happened to the Fat Girl. She didn't just disappear overnight. In fact, I suspect she is still here lurking in the unconscious. She emerges sometimes during that time of the month or when I've had a larger-than-expected gain at Weight Watchers. Her inner critic gets me first and I find myself gripping the steering wheel a little tighter. But I can control her now. And I have a lot more to counter her with, including my new inner Fitness Girl, Fat Girl's alter ego. The Fat Girl doesn't run this body anymore. And perhaps she only remains to serve as a reminder of what could be.

Perhaps that is why I enjoy the mornings as much as I do. That is the time when the Fat Girl is the farthest away from me, even when I am struggling with the morning debate of should I or shouldn't I get up. When I arise in the morning, I know it is something that Fat Girl would never do. She'd stay in bed as long as she could. She didn't want to get up and face the day. But that is precisely what I want to do. My Fitness Girl likes to see the sunrise. She enjoys the feel of exercise and exertion. She doesn't spend too long in front of the mirror and she usually has something in the closet that she is satisfied to wear.

> The Fat Girl doesn't run this body anymore. And perhaps she only remains to serve as a reminder of what could be.

My Fitness Girl can tuck in a shirt if she chooses. She still likes Lucky Charms but eats her low-calorie, high-fiber Puffins Cereal instead. She knows that water is good for her and that cream and sugar are not. She isn't the life of the office anymore. She doesn't gossip nearly as much as she used to; she doesn't make fun of her coworkers behind their backs. But she suspects people like her a little better now than they did before when she had that 30-pound chip on her shoulder.

Fitness Girl still likes fashion just as much my Fat Girl did. That has almost become a dangerous obsession because now she finds herself fitting into the clothing at stores like Banana Republic and the designer boutique at Marshall Field's. Clothing is flattering, too. Even when it comes in colors other than black.

But more important than anything else, the Fitness Girl inside me somehow learned balance. She learned that life wasn't all or nothing.

She could still enjoy food without obsessing over it. She could become fit without spending five hours every day at the gym. She could challenge herself to improve without being hypercritical of every thought or motion. And she also learned about how to enjoy the small things, small things such as her morning ritual. Getting up, working out, cleansing, eating. Life is too short to wake up grumpy and not salute the inner goddess.

That is what Fitness Girl taught Fat Girl. And I'm a better girl for it.

> I never worry about diets. The only carrots that interest me are the number you get in a diamond.
>
> —Mae West

Wrestling Betsy
By Shauna Marsh

I can't remember when I gave my inner Fat Girl a name. But at some point I decided that if I was going to be continually arguing with a voice in my head, I might as well call it Betsy.

Betsy is the one who makes my whole life about the Fat. Sometimes she's a quietly whispered voice in my ear; sometimes she's a destructive, all-powerful force that loves to hold me back and stop me from shining.

Betsy and I go way back. Before I got seriously overweight, she came in the form of typical adolescent angst. All through my teens we'd examine my body from every angle, finding new things to be unhappy about, convincing me I was somehow not up to scratch.

As I grew older and wider, Betsy's voice got louder and more damaging. She took up residence in every extra pound of flesh, to the point where she tainted all my thoughts. I'd be parked on the couch on a Saturday night, mowing my way through a bag of Doritos and asking myself why I kept doing this. Betsy would pipe up, *Well, what else would you be doing? You don't want your friends seeing you like this. No guy is going to be interested. Now, why don't you go fire up the car. I reckon we'll make the McDonald's drive-through before it closes.*

Betsy's most destructive quality is her inferiority complex. She assumes that because I'm fat, I'm stupid. She assumes everyone else knows better just because they're skinny. For years it has been my natural and unthinking response to walk into a room of friends or strangers and assume they're all smarter, funnier, and just plain *better* than I am.

An example of this is how Betsy quietly sabotages my career. There are countless job applications I never made and promotions I never sought because I believed I didn't deserve success. I never piped up in meetings, convinced my opinions were not worth hearing. *Don't say a word*, Betsy would hiss. *Everyone will look at you and all your chins, the way your head just disappears into your shoulders. Do you want twenty people wondering where your neck went?*

If I saw something wrong at work—a colleague's error, a process that could be improved—I'd keep quiet, for my ideas couldn't possibly be valid. If it was really that important, surely someone smarter (and skinnier) would have noticed and done something already?

Good ol' Betsy. She wouldn't let me forget for one second that I was fat and that the fat ruled my life.

It wasn't until I'd lost a good 70 pounds that I started to question her. I'd been going to the gym for about a year, following a program that the gym staff had set for me—treadmill and stationary bike. I was bored and was not seeing any improvement. I read

> Just when you think you've conquered her, when you think your identity is no longer about your lard, Betsy will pop up again.

up on exercise in magazines and online, concluding that weight training would kick-start my weight-loss efforts. But when I asked the gym staff about it, they told me there was no point starting until I got smaller, because lifting would make me heavier and I'd only get discouraged.

All my research told me that that was rubbish, and I knew my body was crying out for a new challenge. But I ignored my gut feeling and listened to Betsy. *What would you know, Shauna? Trust the nubile gym bunnies. How could anyone so toned and blond possibly be wrong?*

So I galumphed along on the treadmill for another two months before finally summoning the courage to trust my own instinct.

My confidence soared as my fitness improved, spilling into other areas of my life. I couldn't believe how much time I'd wasted, how much living I'd missed out on, because of my negative thinking.

Betsy was miffed. She sulked in a dusty corner of my brain while I was busy learning how to think for myself, how to carve out a new identity, how to see myself as a person and not a spineless gimp in a fat suit.

But my girl Betsy is stubborn. Betsy is reluctant to change. No matter how much weight I lose, she always chimes in with her two cents. We argue constantly. A typical exchange:

SHAUNA: That guy is totally checking out my boobs. Cool!
BETSY: Yeah, he's checking out your boobs all right. And thinking how *monstrously flabby* they are!

Just when you think you've conquered her, when you think your identity is no longer about your lard, Betsy will pop up again. At the moment we're debating the merits of running. I am keen to take it up; she thinks it's pointless. *Fat Chicks can't run. Shouldn't you spare the general public the sight of your ungainly, undulating flesh?*

> I don't think I'll ever conquer my inner Fat Girl; I just have to learn to manage her presence.

Today I stood across the street from the running store for fifteen minutes. I needed running shoes, but I was too terrified to step inside. Betsy's old assumptions came flooding back. *You're too fat to go in there. There's no point. You'll never be able to run anyway. Not with this body.* Before long I gave up and went home in tears.

Some days Betsy's voice shouts the loudest.

I don't think I'll ever conquer my inner Fat Girl; I just have to learn to manage her presence. She's like an irritating old friend that you never really liked. Somehow she's got hold of your number and she insists on calling you now and then, just to remind you she's still alive.

You can listen to her ramble for a while—as long as you know when to say, *Shut up, Betsy,* and slam down the phone.

My Fat Girl
By Erin J. Shea

The Fat Girl sits in one of two possible locations in your classroom: the back so no one sees her or in the front because she needs to compensate for her looks by being the smartest one present.

She is the one who hit puberty before everyone else—small mounds of flesh appear on her chest and hips and body overnight—but she continues to share this new body, this *woman's* body, with thick layers of padding left over from her childhood.

The Fat Girl is the teenager who sits at home on the night of the homecoming dance because either no one asked her, or because she was too afraid to go by herself. Maybe she's there, but her date is just a friend. And when Peter Gabriel's "In Your Eyes" streams out from the speakers above, she and her date aren't lost in the pubescent wonder of love and sex with arms tangled lovingly around each other's necks.

They've left the dance floor and are sitting at a table in back talking about algebra class. The Fat Girl is careful not to let her eyes drift over toward her peers as they take part in a mating ritual she dreamed about as a little girl but will clearly never experience herself.

Sometimes, though, she can't help but watch.

Her chief emotion is longing, and as we get older, the Fat Girl is the voice reminding us we are different, not desirable, and certainly not good enough, we are convinced, to handle any situation that a girl with less girth would navigate with ease.

The Fat Girl dictates how we see ourselves.

My Fat Girl is short and awkward, with hair that is always, without fail, down around her face and styled. Her makeup is always applied, nails polished so often that the beds are yellow. My Fat Girl can't get away with the tousled, mussed-up look in public. She knows what people would think of her.

"Look at that lazy fat girl! Doesn't she have *any* shame?"

Her face is so round, it has all the definition of a tomato. My Fat Girl can't remember a time when her inner thighs didn't touch, or that her stomach didn't roll past the top of her pants—especially when she sits down. She never wears patterns of any sort, but she accessorizes with the best of them because the only way she can look trendy is when she's wearing a pair of fancy shoes. Screw Old Navy and Lane Bryant and their tube tops and halters made in larger sizes. My Fat Girl knows that if she even tried to wear such things the stares would be more intense than any trip on the treadmill. My Fat Girl makes self-deprecating remarks in crowded, smoky, noisy bars as her eyes travel over women in tight black pants that sling just below their navels, exposing just a fraction of skin between the pants and the fitted, sleeveless shirt on top. She makes comments about those girls, secretly wishing that she could pull off such a look. Even if she'd never wear a baby tee with the word *Sexy* emblazoned across her tits, she'd at least like to have that option. My Fat Girl remembers how many times she dieted and lost weight in the past. All of the cheerful comments from friends and family members.

"Oh, Erin! When you get to high school all the boys will be after you!"

"Wow, kid! Do you look fantastic!"

"Just look at how much your face has thinned out! And your *thighs!*"

She usually remembers these things as she is stripping every last piece of clothing from her closet, looking for something—anything— that fits without having to grab her sewing kit to move that button over just an inch more. Even if those methods of Diets Past left her weak and frail, they obviously left her more attractive.

My Fat Girl has stopped even pretending that anyone would ever find her attractive, even though enough men have told her that she's beautiful. Enough that she almost believed them. And those men, at one point, loved her very much.

But she never believed them. She could never believe it herself.

My Fat Girl dreams about running in a race. My Fat Girl dreams about having arms protruding with more muscle than they do fat. My Fat Girl dreams about pants with a motherfucking belt. Not even a fancy belt! Just a belt . . . and maybe a shirt tucked in for good measure.

She has sat in her living room with a hot, brown paper bag filled to the brim with a super-sized fry and a cheeseburger. A lone cherry pie congealed with grease at the bottom of it all. My Fat Girl has spent an entire day with her head buried deep in a carton of ice cream. She has eaten a family-sized bag of Cheetos, taking nary a breath before she grabs the pretzels.

Pretzels are a poor substitute, but they are the only thing left that will do.

My Fat Girl has been alone, wishing someone would just make it all go away.

Such a way of living has not been my reality in years, yet I can't escape the memory of what those binges did to me.

> My Fat Girl has spent an entire day with her head buried deep in a carton of ice cream. She has eaten a family-sized bag of Cheetos, taking nary a breath before she grabs the pretzels.

No matter my achievements both personally and professionally, no matter if people no longer consider me fat, if I'm not even fat at all, I am still this Fat Girl.

Nearly every woman has struggled with her body in one way or another and for some, rarely have they known an identity for themselves beyond their bodies. The Fat Girl is the amalgamation of traditional adolescence angst and of being picked last, or never being chosen at all, one too many times. I've yet to find a woman who doesn't have a Fat Girl living inside her.

After losing weight, I hoped the Fat Girl would go away. When someone brings doughnuts into the office, would I once again hear her telling me to wait until the coast is clear before even grabbing a plain, nonglazed variety, or could I join the morning rush without fear?

Could I walk into a restaurant and not think its patrons were scrutinizing my outfit, let alone me? Could I eat a meal and not consider the effect of its caloric content and whether or not I had time to work off anything extra?

But, she hasn't gone anywhere.

I took a kickboxing class once, and despite knowing that I kicked some major boxing butt, I worried for the entire duration of the class that when I was complimented on my work, it was because the instructor was so happy that the Fat Girl was giving it her all.

I'm starting to come to the conclusion that my Fat Girl may just be around for good.

But I'm also beginning to have some peace with her. Though, now she is only a part of me. Instead of dictating my every move, holding me hostage, my Fat Girl is much like the family member who never lets you forget where you came from no matter how successful you become.

My Fat Girl is a little happier these days. She's beginning to see a life beyond being fat. Oh, sure, she still wants a super-sized fry every blessed day—and sometimes I indulge her—but she's getting used to pita and hummus. Some days she tries to talk me into hitting the snooze button on gym mornings; my Fat Girl wins this battle once in a while, so I try to catch her off guard later and hit the treadmill when she's not looking.

Despite all of this, my Fat Girl figures the hummus alone is worth it; after all, we may not have conquered all of our demons, and we're not perfect, but we look fabulous in a belt.

The Devil Inside
By Robyn Anderson

My inner Fat Girl resembles Mimi from *The Drew Carey Show*. Okay, she doesn't resemble her—she's a dead ringer for her. The weird, wild clothes, the crazy makeup, and the voice—good lord, the voice. She could conquer countries once she gets going with that voice. Is it any wonder that when she starts whining for a dozen Krispy Kremes to ram down our throat I'm tempted to go out and buy the damn things? Just to shut her up?

I call her Tallulah, and she's a total drama queen, my inner Fat Girl. Everything's black and white, with no in-betweens. To her, life is summed up by two simple equations:

- Exercise and salads = ick!
- Sugar and crappy junk food = yum!

I don't know how long she's been there in my head, making my life miserable, but I'd hazard a guess that she was created when I was young and chubby, and as I got older and fatter she got stronger and louder. Every time someone made a comment about my weight, every time some asshole drove by and mooed at me, every time I thought that the only important thing about me was that number on the scale, every time I realized anew that I couldn't fit into the clothes from the "normal people" store, every time I caught a sidelong glance from a stranger and was immediately made aware that I was seen as lazy and smelly and stupid because of my size, my inner Fat Girl grew and grew and grew. She took up more space in my brain, sounding more assured, as if every word she spoke were the truth, until I took every word she said as gospel.

And my inner Fat Girl is *such* a bitch.

"Are you going to wear *that*? Don't you know how fat you are? Don't you know *you* can't wear something like that? Don't you know how horrible you'll look, and people will turn and stare? Let's just stay home and eat. Let's sit on the couch in front of the television. Oh, *fuck* that exercising stuff. You haven't lost weight in more months than I can count. What's the point? It's no *fun*. Let's eat, let's eat, *let's eat*."

The one thing that actually shuts her up? Food. I can get her to be quiet for a while by exercising hard, but I can only lift weights or do cardio for so long. Sooner or later I have to rest, and then she starts up again with her relentless banter.

She's even worse in places where food is immediately available. If I walk through the grocery store, she's like a two-year-old, yelling, "Oooh! Cake! Let's get cake! Ooh! Candy! Me want candy!" My willpower and I counter every demand with a simple, firm "Uh, *no*," but she never quite shuts up. "Bagels! Muffins! Candy! *Candy! Candy!*" She's a bit of a sugar freak. Don't try to pacify her with a salad or fruit or yogurt or anything with the slightest bit of redeeming nutritional value. She wants sugar and cake and cookies, and she wants them *now*. When I go out to eat at a restaurant, she doesn't even want to wait until the main course gets there—she wants a basket of bread or some huge appetizer, and she's willing to have a screaming fit if she doesn't get her way.

> My inner Fat Girl is *such* a bitch.

She loves to make me self-conscious about the way my shirts ride up in the front. She yells "Pull your shirt *down*. Pull your shirt away from your body. People will see that you're fat!" I'm not sure who she thinks she's kidding, because I have a feeling people will know I'm fat whether my shirt touches my body or not.

91

Sometimes I try to visualize her away. I think of her as the devil, squatting on one shoulder, whispering evil things in my ear. Her nemesis—the inner Skinny Angel—sits on the other, buff from working out and ready to walk across my back to put my inner Fat Chick out of my misery. Since the Skinny Angel is so very buff (half an hour on the elliptical trainer *without* stopping to catch her breath, you know), one would expect her to make short work of the devil, but that inner Fat Chick of mine is more tenacious than you'd expect. All she has to do is hold on and kick really hard, and the Skinny Angel hasn't got a chance.

I don't know if it's possible, after she's lived in my head more than twenty-five years, to ever completely get rid of her. I can always feel her hovering nearby, waiting to judge me and what I eat ("Ugh, *salad*? No fun!"), radiating disapproval when I decide to do forty minutes on the elliptical trainer instead of thirty, or putting on a shirt that comes close to fitting instead of being three sizes too big.

One would think that with weight loss would come a quieting of her voice, but it seems that she doesn't care what I actually weigh. I've lost 125 pounds? She doesn't care. She doesn't care about the reality, just what she decided years ago is the truth, and she wants to yell her truth from the mountaintop. I am fat and disgusting, and anyone who makes a snide comment about my weight gets a pat on the back because they're only speaking the truth—and you can't be mad at people for speaking the truth, can you?

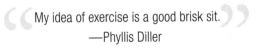

My idea of exercise is a good brisk sit.
—Phyllis Diller

Whisper to a Scream
By Lori Ford

I think it's every Fat Girl's dream to just be accepted for who they are. My body and my clothes are forever changing. I've bought every size at the Gap and my limited time in Lane Bryant is more than enough. And no matter what I'm wearing or what size I am, I'm still the same person on the inside. I have the same hopes and dreams, the same sense of humor, the same likes and dislikes. It's a fact, however, that I'm treated differently based on whatever size I may be.

My self-esteem and my body image are fused together. They are not supposed to be. You're supposed to be able to separate how you feel about your body and how you feel about yourself as a person. You're supposed to be able to be overweight and not let it affect your mood or your personality. It doesn't work that way for me.

Thin equals beautiful and beautiful equals perfection. I've grown up with this imbedded in me. Every time I try to forget it, someone or something will remind me. Society makes it abundantly clear what it caters to.

While I was growing up, I was never allowed to develop my personality. I was expected to do what I was told and never complain, be polite and courteous and unselfish (though I was told I was selfish all the time), and mostly to be quiet and well behaved. I was naturally shy, so most of this was never a problem. In social situations I was to be quiet, quietly drawing, quietly listening, quietly bored. I never recall anyone asking my opinion about anything or being a part of conversations. I didn't really mind, being shy made it uncomfortable to be the center of attention, but at the same time I never really had the chance to work on developing my social skills.

Because I was expected to be quiet and well mannered, I looked to other ways to foster attention. To be recognized. To be loved. I loved to swim and tried to make people notice how good a swimmer I was. I ate up compliments: "You're such a frog, such a good swimmer." I loved to draw and would be tragically disappointed if my pictures weren't recognized, at school, at home, wherever. I remember we had a news station that showed children's drawings during the weather forecast. I remember my picture being on the show. I still remember that. I was desperate to do well in school. I always tested way above average in elementary school.

I also remember getting complimented on my looks. How pretty I was. How angelic. How princesslike. People would look at me and smile. Their faces would soften and their voices would lighten. I wanted to be a princess. Everyone would like me. Everyone would think I was perfect. Quiet. And beautiful. I thought this was perfection because it was what was expected of me.

> No matter what I'm wearing or what size I am, I'm still the same person on the inside. I have the same hopes and dreams, the same sense of humor, the same likes and dislikes.

Then I began to notice I wasn't the prettiest. Girls in school and in ballet were thinner than I was. They had straight legs and mine were curvy. They seemed more poised, more delicate, more graceful. They were also self-confident and articulate. I felt highly inadequate, even at a young age. I was never fat that I can recall and certainly can't tell from pictures, but I was taunted and teased in my late elementary years into middle school. I began to lie even lower so I wouldn't draw attention to myself. I shut down my personality even more.

This is how I think I aligned my overweight body with being less of a person. My personality didn't help me in social situations. I did my best to be quiet and not express myself. Thin meant I was beautiful and beautiful meant I was perfect. Perfection gave me love, attention, and acceptance. Feeling love, attention, and acceptance made me feel better about myself and my self-esteem flourished. At least until the weight came back on, and it always came back on.

Once I was in my preteens everything changed. My mother and father divorced and my mother remarried. She married a very boisterous man with two boisterous sons. At first this helped me. I was the only girl so I was given attention for that reason. The prettier I could appear would give me more attention, from my stepfather and from my brothers. But mostly I was ignored. Time with family was about being boisterous and funny and having things to say. I didn't know what I felt and what I had to say, so I was quiet. Everything seemed to always be happening around me. I was never really part of it. Soon my brother was born and all attention seemed to recede. My brother got everything. I was entering puberty and my weight was problematic. My brothers still had attention because they were loud and had terrific strong personalities. I envied how they had things to say and how they were funny and fun to be around. If I were pretty, they would certainly want to play with me. If I were ugly, certainly they would not. It was also around this time as puberty hit that I naturally began to rebel. I would shut down when I was confronted, and finally one day my mom yelled at me, "Why don't you ever yell back? Yell back at me!" And it was then, in that moment, that I was given permission to express myself, and even though it was in a negative way, it still allowed me to free my inner self.

My mother still tells me to this day how one of my stepbrothers once said if you're thin, you can get away with being a bitch—people will overlook it. If you're fat, you can't. I've spent years losing my anger and don't consider myself a bitch, but I do recognize what's being implied. If you are beautiful (which of course equals thin), you can have personality flaws and still be accepted. If you are fat, you can't. I have lived both lives, as beautiful and as fat, and I would have to say in all honesty, my brother is right.

It's no wonder I feel so messed up. Especially considering I'm never the same weight. I've never really gotten a chance to feel comfortable in my own skin. I don't know who I am outside my weight. If I attend a family function and I'm thin, it's exciting and everyone is smiling and so happy for me. I soak it in and feel happy and excited and, in turn, they think I've had this huge personality breakthrough.

If I attend the same type of function overweight, I panic about it before I even get there. Everyone's going to know I failed at keeping my body. I won't feel good in my own skin and therefore I won't feel good about myself. The smiles won't be as wide and the excitement will be downplayed, and I'll take it to heart, further thinking I've failed. It's no wonder I want to hide in a corner or just go home. I'm quieter and smile less. I keep to myself, trying to hide my failure.

I've spent a lot of time working on my self-esteem while trying to lose weight. Losing weight becomes a pilgrimage. Every focus is on the pilgrimage and what the pilgrimage will bring. The hunger pains and the dreaded doom of exercise are not only tolerable but also expected. I leave behind my old life and its old problems to seek out this magic place called 130 pounds, where self-esteem is ever so abundant. I've trained myself to think that fat means no self-esteem and thin means all is right with the world.

And yet even when I'm thin, my inner Fat Chick will still whisper in my ear, telling me how I have nothing to say, I have nothing to contribute, and they're only interested because I'm beautiful. Which leads to self-doubt, which leads to chocolate cravings, and you understand how that goes.

Fat Girls' Clubhouse

By Monique van den Berg

$\mathcal{T}$he Fat Girl. Close your eyes and picture her.

Is it the Jolly Fat Girl? She's laughing just a little too loudly, the center of attention. She's the one who will be the first to remark on her big ass or her flabby arms. "What a great attitude she has," people say. "She never lets anything get her down."

What about the Sexy Fat Girl? She's wearing that halter top that's just a little too bright and a little too tight. She's overaccessorized. She's making the most of those great tits she has: her favorite compensation for being fat. She's a flirt. She's wearing high-heeled thigh-high boots. She's a fantastic kisser.

Maybe it's the Bitter Fat Girl. She has so many defenses; she's like a fortress of fat guarded by a moat of bitterness full of chocolate-covered sharks. Every time you look at her, she imagines what you must be thinking. If you smile, you're mocking her. If you frown, you're judging her. She tells you to go fuck yourself because she doesn't care what you think about her. Except that she does.

Or the Invisible Fat Girl. She knows she isn't worthy of your notice. She is an expert at looking down, averting her eyes, avoiding the crowd. She is constantly braced for someone to yell, "Hey Fatso!"—as if they're telling her something she doesn't know. She wonders what people whisper about her when she walks by. What they say behind her back.

How about the Less Fat Girl? She walks into a room and hopes she's less fat than the other people in it. She feels superior when this turns out to be the case. She feels great about herself. And this would be okay except that she's also the More Fat Girl. Sometimes she walks into a room and she *is* the fattest person in it. Then she hates herself. They're all better than her because they're all skinnier than she is.

The Girl of Fat Sisterhood. She feels vaguely distrustful of the thin. They have a key to a clubhouse, a way of life that she's excluded from. They know the secrets of the thin. They know what it's like to look at yourself naked and like what you see. She doesn't have that. Her true friends are the Fat Girls. She can let her guard down in front of them. They encourage each other to go out and have some ice cream, some French fries.

The Fat Friend is different. She's the girl in the movies who is best friends with the thin, perky heroine. Her job is to go shopping with Ashley or Britney or Cassidy and sit outside the dressing room, not trying on anything herself (she wouldn't fit into these clothes anyway) and telling Ashley that *of course* those pants don't make her look fat. Her job is to say, "Oh yeah, he's totally into you. Do you want me to go give him your number?" and not to be a threat. Of course, she's not a threat. The Fat Friend never gets the guy.

There's the Worried Fat Girl. She worries about the things that nobody else worries about. Fitting inside the booth at dinner. Being too fat for the amusement park rides.

Of course, I know these Fat Girls. I *am* these Fat Girls. I've spent my whole life being them, one after another, making my identity out of little pieces of each of them. I'm new things and greater things and entirely different things. The Beautiful Fat Girl. The More-Than-Her-Fat Girl. The Quit Trying to Define Me, Damnit, Fat Girl.

And of course, what I'm trying to be: the Former Fat Girl. The Hidden Fat Girl. The Ex-Fat Girl. Who is she? What does she look like? Is she lurking inside, waiting to take over? Will she be happy, healthy, whole?

Will she miss the fat that once defined her?

Will she know who she is without it?

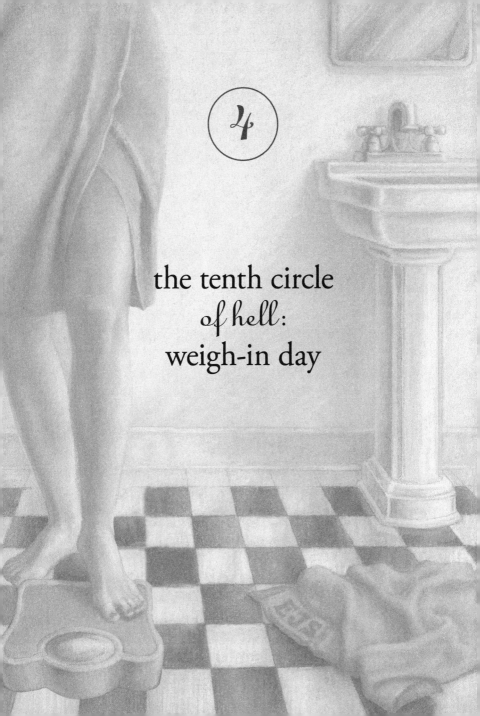

4

the tenth circle
of hell:
weigh-in day

I Have to Get Up:
I Have to Go to the Gym.

It's only six. I can sleep another fifteen minutes and still get up and still go to the gym and still work out and still take a shower and still get into the car and still get onto the bus and still get to work on time.

Whatever. Maybe I'll just sleep in. I went yesterday.

I have to get up. I'll just do twenty minutes of cardio. And crunches, I guess. If I get up in five minutes I can maybe do those. My abs are looking pretty good, actually, and I think if I do eighty today then maybe this weekend I can do a hundred.

Ten more minutes. Does it even matter if I work out? I seem to have *gained* weight in the past couple of weeks, going three times a week, and I was staying the same when I was only going twice a week. Is working out making me fat?

Fatter, I mean. It totally doesn't matter if I work out if I'm just going to get fatter. I'm totally sleeping in and I'm never going to the gym again because the gym is *stupid* and I *hate* it. *Hate* the gym.

By Chiara LaRotonda

If I'm trying to lose weight, am I totally giving in to the man? I mean, the Man? Am I buying into unrealistic media-fueled expectations about women's bodies that I can't conceivably live up to? And how come that endorphin high I keep hearing about never happens to me? I *hate* the gym.

Of course, there is that whole diabetes-on-both-sides-of-the-family thing. So I should definitely go, and I am going. I'm going in just five more minutes.

If I have to ask for a size 16 one more time at Old Navy, I think I will lie down on the floor and cry. I have to get up.

Where are my yoga pants? Dryer? Living-room floor? Still in the gym bag?

I guess I could just go today after work and still sleep a little more.

I could have been up and in the car and on the treadmill by now instead of arguing with myself. I could be there right now and then I would be done in twenty minutes and then I could be showering and getting dressed and walking out the door at 7:30 with a *stunning* feeling of self-righteousness. I could be at work right this minute, with my hair wet and going casually, "Oh, yeah, I *went to the gym* this morning." Yet, I am still in bed and I have to get up and I'm going to be late even if I *don't* go into the gym, but if I'm going to be late anyway, I might as well, and I don't know where my yoga pants are and I don't know where my nonyoga pants are but I have to go, have to go, have to go.

Now. Right now.

Fuggedabouit
By Julie Ridl

Okay, listen up: It's not about the damned scale.

The scale is not a slot machine. It does not steal, nor does it pay off.

The scale provides one small measure of your fitness progress, and not a very good one.

The scale doesn't care if you have your period and are carrying extra fluid.

The scale doesn't care if you're a little sensitive to the MSG you ate that bloated your bod.

The scale doesn't care how hard you worked out this week, how sore you are, and how much water your sore muscles are holding.

The scale doesn't know you've been ill.

The scale doesn't know you're constipated.

The scale doesn't know you've been working out hard and have developed muscles.

The scale doesn't know you've been heavy for a long time and carry heavy muscles and denser bones than when you were twelve.

No.

No, no, no, no, no.

The scale doesn't know you, love you, or hate you.

It doesn't recognize you. It doesn't see you coming.

It is not your friend; it is not your enemy.

It is not kind to you one week and cruel you the next.

It has no life or conscience at all. It is a measuring device, and the only thing it measures is your total weight at the moment you step on it.

The number it reveals? That number is the combined total of your present lean body weight, fat weight, and the enormously variable amount of fluid (water weight) healthy bodies carry around. It doesn't measure mass. And reducing your fat mass is all you're after. That and reducing your blood pressure, getting your blood sugar under control, reducing your blood cholesterol, your resting heart rate.

Here's a radical idea: Your total body weight doesn't matter. It's only the amount of your fat, and whether it's within a healthy range, that matters.

A girlfriend who's working out hard at Curves and watching her food carefully told me yesterday her scale wasn't budging. She's buff, she's gorgeous, and she just threw out some khakis that are now too big for her, but the scale isn't budging. So what?

> The scale is not a slot machine. It does not steal, nor does it pay off.

A buddy on a Web board yesterday said she was "scared to get on the scale" yesterday, but did and saw she'd lost a pound last week. So, she thinks she'll stick with her program after all.

And if that scale hadn't registered a drop? I'm saying she was ready to restore all of her old, unhealthy habits based on what that scale read.

There is so much that I adore about Weight Watchers, but I'd just give anything for those folks to redesign the meetings and requirements and training to de-emphasize the weigh-in.

It's just not that important.

What's important? Developing new habits is important. Exploring healthier foods and learning to cook them and like them is important. Eating smaller meals is important. Making exercise a habit is important. Tracking energy in and energy out by writing down what you eat and how much you exercise, that's important.

I'm looking for the program that has no mandatory weigh-in, but has mandatory journal-keeping as its threshold for weekly meetings. I'm looking for the program that gives people gold stars and stickers not for weight loss, but for increasing their weight or reps on the leg-press machine, or walking a half mile every day, or trying bok choy and learning that cabbage can too be delicious and satisfying.

How about a sticker for bringing in an interesting nutrition article?

How about a sticker for helping out a fellow loser who's feeling down?

How about a sticker for not eating in front of the TV at night?

Forget the damned scale. Put it away. Don't fear it. Don't think about it. Think instead about what you're doing. If you're staying on your program, then you're succeeding. If you're not, then figure out what you need to do to get back on program again. If you know you've been good, then feel good. You're a winner.

If it's been three or four weeks and your jeans aren't any looser? Then modify your program to reduce your food intake and step up your workouts. Follow that for three more weeks, and check to see how your jeans fit again.

I'm saying, it's not a numbers game. Instead, pick a dress size, pick a suit jacket size as your goal. Pick a blood lipid number, a blood pressure reading, a resting heart rate goal.

And for crying out loud, be patient! It takes awhile for your complex and miraculously designed body to respond to all the new signals you're giving it.

Consider this: It's possible to lose weight and get fit without any scales at all.

The Scale

By Heather Lockwood

We are so focused on numbers. In the weight-loss world, we cannot escape them. We measure our body fat. We feel judged by our clothing size. There are the inches around our waists and necks and calves to be tallied. And there is the number on the scale, the supreme number that rules all.

These numbers in and of themselves don't mean a whole lot. After all, they are just that: numbers. They are arbitrary digits that fluctuate and change and differ from person to person. But these numbers are our only concrete means for measurement. In a clinical setting, they are the only way to measure progress. Therefore, they have a hold over us that is sometimes inescapable and often maddening.

In many ways, these numbers make up who I am, much like a portfolio. They generate my self-worth. They tell me if I am good or bad or mediocre. And the outside world confirms this.

Blood pressure: 120 / 70. *Good girl, perfect.*

Red blood cell count: 34. *Bad girl, a little low. Are you getting enough iron?*

Weight: 145. *That's a little high.*

Resting heart rate: 45. *Excellent health.*

Waist: 28 inches. *Good. Nice.*

Hips: 48 inches. *Hmmm . . . A few two many slices of cheesecake, eh?*

Body fat percentage: *28 percent. Oh, that should be a little lower for optimum health.*

Yet what does all this tell you about me, really? Does this give you a picture of who I really am? Does this tell you that I'm a Democrat or a Republican? Do these numbers indicate whether or not I have children? Can you tell if I volunteer or donate to charity? Do you know what car I drive?

I've gotten to that point in the Weight Watchers program where I need to declare a goal, a numeric goal. I can no longer use the vague statement, "I just want to lose some weight and be healthy." Not if I want to become a lifetime member, at least. I'm getting close to my goal range, or better yet, "Weight Watchers' goal range" for my height and age. At this stage in the process, they want me to pinpoint a number on the scale that will represent the perfect me. Yet, I feel a little helpless because I don't know what that is.

I have spent years focusing on that number on the scale. My very first driver's license issued was a lie. Even then, I felt the need to drop an extra 5 pounds when committing the scale number to paper. For some reason, 125 seemed like such a better weight than 130. Of course, had I been 125 at the time, I'd bet I would have dropped that number even lower. Which is really crazy. Who looks at the number on a person's driver license besides that person anyway? I thought I was putting that false number on there to hide my weight from the world. In actuality, I was merely hiding the truth from myself.

> I've never owned a scale. I think that is really odd for someone who has spent the better part of her thirty-two years obsessed with her weight.

I've never owned a scale. I think that is really odd for someone who has spent the better part of her thirty-two years obsessed with her weight. I don't know if the reasoning behind this is that I've been cheap or I just didn't want to face the truth in the confines of my bathroom. Because I've never owned a scale myself, I'm a whore when it comes to scales in other places. If I'm in the bathroom at a dinner party at a friend's home and I notice a scale pushed off to the side, I'll pull it out and weigh myself. If I'm at the grocery store and they have one of those twenty-five-cent weight-and-fortune machines, I'll insert my quarter. I've even been known to pull a scale off the shelf at Target. If anyone asks, I'm just testing.

Subconsciously, I think I do all this on purpose. All these arbitrary weigh-ins in all these arbitrary places occur because they never really count, not in my mind. Because they never occur at a consistent time and place, I am able to rationalize why the number that appears is not ideal. My head can knock out justifications left and right: *The pants I'm wearing are heavy. I just ate a large meal. It is that time of the month.*

I've spent years never really knowing what I weighed because I couldn't face the truth that these guerrilla-style weigh-ins were telling me. And since I didn't have a scale at home, I never had to confirm it.

The day that I first discovered that I had nudged into the 170s, I was in my mother's upstairs bathroom. I had just finished washing my hands and reapplying my lip-gloss and I spotted the scale pushed off to the side. I pulled it out, stepped on top, and as the number started to bounce between 165 and 172, I stepped off immediately, not wanting to face the truth. I couldn't possibly weigh that much. Not me.

A couple of weeks later, I was at the grocery store. This time, partly out of curiosity and partly in an attempt to erase the event in my mother's bathroom, I inserted a quarter into the weight-and-fortune machine. When I saw 172 in red digital letters, it made me slightly ill. But it wasn't until it was printed on the little slip of paper with my fortune attached that it really hit home: 172, my highest weight ever. I crumpled up the paper and threw it in the trash. I didn't even read my fortune. I didn't have to.

For the next year or so, I avoided this number. My scale hit-and-runs came to a halt because my suspicion was that nothing much had changed. I wasn't losing weight and I didn't want a reminder that

I weighed nearly as much as my husband. I didn't want to know for sure that I had gained a good 35 pounds since college. And I didn't want to have to face the knowledge that my weight was pushing my health into dangerous territories. After all, I didn't feel that unhealthy. My husband told me I looked pretty. I didn't feel overweight.

By now I started a nearly scale-free existence. It was almost liberating. Had it not been for the fact that the extra poundage was starting to affect other aspects of my life, I would probably have never weighed myself again for the rest of my life. I didn't need that stress of having to live my life on the basis of some arbitrary number.

Of course, the weight began to speak to me in other ways. If I couldn't take the hint from the scale, I eventually had to take it from the size of my pants and my fitness level. At a point of enlightenment, I joined a gym and started working out. The extra pounds started to come off and I began at some point to face the scale again.

Of course, this time I did it with purpose. In addition to my scale pop-ons in the homes of my friends, I started a regular weigh-in day where I kept all variables the same. Each Wednesday after working out, showering, and releasing my bladder, I'd step onto the digital scale, flip-flops off, with one white towel wrapped around my midsection. And for the first time in my life, I started to keep track of my progress. The scale that I had liberated myself from had once again taken a role of judgment in my life. Only this time I felt I had more control.

This was the routine that saw me through the vast majority of my weight loss. I never had any concrete goals in mind. I only wanted the number on the scale to go down. I refused to make things more concrete than that. Then one day the number on the scale stopped moving and I once again liberated myself from its grasp.

I had hit the upper 140s, although I really came to a rest at 150 pounds. After losing as much as 30 pounds from my highest weight,

I was proud of how far I'd come. I knew that eventually I'd like to lose more, but it was no longer a priority. My health was finally in order and I was sick of having to weigh in each week only to be let down because I didn't see any progress in those red digital numbers. Besides, there was progress in other areas that meant much more than that damn scale could ever compete with. I'd run my first 5k. I'd completed a triathlon. There was a century bike ride, too. If the scale wasn't telling me what I wanted to hear, my fitness was.

Then, one February afternoon, I received an e-mail at work. It advertised my company's Weight Watchers at Work program and I was curious. In the past, I had made fun of friends who participated in Weight Watchers because they were essentially paying to weigh in, something I figured could be done for free. I didn't understand the concept. But I couldn't dispute the fact that I had also seen many friends find success with the program. And since I still wasn't exactly where I wanted to be, I figured it was worth a try. If nothing more, I would find out what all the fuss was about.

Right off the bat, I started losing weight. I couldn't believe it. Much of this progress was due to the modified eating plan. But I also felt a certain responsibility when I knew I was paying to weigh in. I hated the fact that this worked, but I enjoyed it, too. Soon, I was at my lowest weight since college.

Of course, now, eighteen weeks later, I've found myself in unknown territory. I'm dangerously close to being done. I'm also dangerously close to giving up. I haven't picked a goal and I don't know what it should be.

I've accomplished so much with my struggles with weight. I've even overcome my aversion to the scale. When I weighed in two weeks ago, I had hit 141 pounds. For my height and weight, that is the topmost number in my healthy body range. I could stop here if I wanted. The leader asked me when she wrote down this number, "So? Is this it?"

"I don't know," was all I could answer. "I'm not sure. Should it be? I don't want to make this too hard and set a goal of something I can't maintain."

"You don't want to sell yourself short, either" was her response as she slipped my weight log back into its plastic sleeve. "You have to make the decision as to what is right for you. Let me know when you know."

And since then, I've been in limbo. I'm suddenly faced with the question, "Am I happy where I am?" And I'm not sure. I think I am. I like the way I look. But I'd also like to be skinnier. I just don't know.

At the end of the day, I know it is not the number on the scale that will determine my success. The ultimate measure will be how I feel on the inside and out. Unfortunately, that feeling isn't something that can be logged by Weight Watchers or by my doctor. They need something more concrete than that. They need a number, something a scale can provide, which serves as a symbol of progress. It is the best they can do.

So when I think about my goal, I need to look at it in those terms. It is just a symbol, something that can be measured. It is just part of a greater whole. I've spent too long working hard with no finish line in sight. I'm ready to turn the corner and see it. I'm ready to finish those last few steps. I'm ready to make a goal.

I've fought against confining my self-worth to a number on a scale my entire life. I know what constitutes my health is much greater than that. But I've also come to the realization that I do need goals. And if setting a number on the scale can help me accomplish that, then that is what I need to do. So, there you go. I'm ready to put a number on paper. That kind of feels good.

The Trouble with Mirrors
By Shauna Marsh

℮ xercise is like sex. If you thought about what you looked like while you're doing it, you wouldn't do it at all.

For the longest time I worried about what I looked like, so I didn't get much. Exercise, that is. The idea of moving my 350-pound frame in any fashion was horrifying. I got red-faced and puffed from making my bed and walking to the fridge, let alone from formal exercise. And exercise usually involves some sort of public humiliation. When you're obese, you devote your energy to moving your bulk as little as possible, in order to minimize the attention drawn to it.

For the first few months of my weight-loss journey I focused entirely on changing my eating habits. Lifting vegetables to my mouth instead of chocolate was exertion enough. But when my loss started to slow down on the scale, I knew I'd have to take things up a notch if I wanted it to continue.

I started out with walking the dog. I figured this was the least mortifying option. I could either go early in the morning or just as night fell, so the crowds and temperature would be minimal. At first I could only galumph along helplessly as Harry hauled me down to the end of the block. Then I had to stop and clutch my knees and wait for my heart to stop thumping against my rib cage. Then I'd catch sight of my reflection in a car window and want to cry. Why did I pick such a small dog from the shelter? I should have got a huge slobbering Saint Bernard; at least we'd be more in proportion. As soon as Harry was done pissing on the tires, I'd turn around and go home.

Total workout time: ten minutes.

But I persisted. Eventually we made it all the way around the block. Every few weeks I'd add on another block, then another. Then a whole extra street.

Soon I felt confident enough to scrape the dust off my membership card and venture back into the gym. I tried out the treadmill, the bike, and the elliptical machine; each contraption seemed designed to find new and unflattering ways to redistribute my bulk. Multitudes of mirrors captured it from every angle, with crop-topped blonds running around in the background to kill any dying embers of self-esteem.

In spite of that, I persevered. My weight continued to drop and my fitness improved, but I found exercise to be a tiresome chore. The experts say you need to exercise at least three times a week. Would I have to be this *bloody bored* at least three times a week for the rest of my life?

I vowed to experiment until I found My Exercise. I endured ten minutes of an aerobics video until I flopped on the couch to glare at the perky instructor. Same thing happened with the yoga show on cable TV. I even tried swimming but only got as far as the foyer before I panicked and fled at the idea of unveiling my pale, dimpled flesh.

Finally, ten months into my weight-loss journey, I struck gold. I'd been curious about the mysterious room at the end of the gym, where you could hear the faint thump *thump, thump* of dance music and catch glimpses of grunting sweaty bodies through the little window. No, it wasn't the set of a porn movie—it was the aerobics studio.

It was like I'd found the door to Narnia in the back of my closet. That first Body Pump changed my whole attitude toward exercise and gave me hope that I could actually *enjoy* moving my lardy ass. It was one hour of free weights accompanied by rocking tunes. I hid in the back row and fumbled with the equipment and *loved it*.

Body Pump combined my love of music and laziness. All I had to do was show up and some athletic wench would yell and scream and tell me exactly how to move my butt. The next day my muscles screamed, but I knew I'd done more for my weight-loss campaign in that hour than during months of directionless cavorting on the machines.

An addiction was born. I tried spinning, kickboxing, yoga, tai chi, and dancing. I'd been overweight and then obese for close to a decade, so I didn't know much about fitness, I didn't know diddly-squat about squats. So the class format suited me well. I got motivation and education from the instructors and relaxation from the music. At first I felt embarrassed, being so much larger than my classmates, but soon I realized they were all in their own little worlds, focusing on their own bodies. My classes became a haven where I could be part of a group, yet disappear quietly into my own mind. I'd ponder my weight-loss efforts, compose shopping lists, or think deep thoughts like *One more squat and everyone's gonna know I ate chili con carne for dinner.*

During exercise, I'd ponder my weight-loss efforts, compose shopping lists, or think deep thoughts like *One more squat and everyone's gonna know I ate chili con carne for dinner.*

My weight loss accelerated and my body began to take shape beneath the blubber. I'd lie in the dark at night, poking and prodding my new muscles. Everyday life was easier; I no longer panicked at a flight of stairs or if a colleague asked me along for a walk to the mall at lunchtime.

But the mental changes were the most dramatic. Instead of seeing my body as useless and ugly, I started to feel pride in what it was now capable of, how it grew stronger and fitter every day. My moods improved so much I no longer needed my depression medication.

One scorching December day in Australia, eleven months into my journey, I rocked up to the gym to find it was closed due to a maintenance issue. I stomped back to the car, flung my backpack into the backseat, then pounded the steering wheel. How dare they! How dare they cancel *my* class! I fumed for a good five minutes before catching my stormy expression in the rearview mirror. I had to laugh. Somehow, in under a year, I'd transformed from couch slug to chronic gym rage.

These days, I don't worry about what I look like in the mirrors at the gym. I screw up, I trip over, but now I can just laugh about it. And it helps to notice that other people screw up, too. Even skinny people can be clumsy! But we're all there, people of all shapes and sizes and skill levels, for the love of moving our asses. Exercise is fundamentally a sweaty and silly pursuit, but don't it feel so good?

Like I said before, it's just like sex.

> I have gained and lost the same ten pounds so many times over and over again, my cellulite must have déjà vu.
>
> —Jane Wagner

Overflow
By Erin J. Shea

Wait.

185?

Let's try that again.

Deep breath. Suck in the gut, as if somehow sucking in your gut magically sends the weight to a faraway land, like when you take a picture and somehow weighing in on a scale is like a snapshot in time, right? Right. Gingerly touch the scale with your right foot. Follow similarly with the left. Stand erect.

182?

That can't be right either.

Move scale. Closer to the bathroom shower. Brace self against wall, careful not to knock over any of the assorted knickknacks adorning your toilet. Grasp the side of the shower stall, with a similar amount of care as to not fall face-first into the door. Tiptoe up to the edge of the scale, still bracing wall while simultaneously holding onto stall door, and shift weight as you watch the numbers climb. And climb.

Stop.

Situate body so that your right hip is resting against the door, placing the majority of your weight on that door, but all the while bracing the remainder of your weight against the wall, and for Christ's sake, don't let go of the stall! Balance on one foot, preferably the right one. Look down at scale. Pray.

123.

That sounds right.

Get off scale. Return to kitchen. Pretend you had stomach cramps when someone asks you what took so long. Eat a Ho-Ho. Be amazed that you're officially fat. Eat another one.

They do not let you do that shit at Weight Watchers.

At Weight Watchers, you have to step up on a scale that is a miniature replica of the scales I assume are used for livestock at the county fair. There is no escaping the accuracy with which these scales measure weight and they certainly don't allow for the wink and a smile that a medical scale allows. The scale in a doctor's office allows a person to trick herself into believing her weight isn't actually what it is. Those little lines in between the numbers are symbolic of an *actual* number, I know, but because there isn't a number present, those lines give me permission to pretend I am a better weight. A good weight! A weight that behaves and covers its mouth when it burps and never sneaks a second helping of potatoes.

I *might* be 175 pounds, but clearly the lever isn't convinced enough with that number that it balances out. It sways up and down, undecided. Had it rested squarely upon 175, I'd then have to flail my arms about and complain. Since it can't make a decision, as far as I'm concerned, I weigh anywhere between 115 to 170 pounds.

On a scale at Weight Watchers, those lines turn into the cold, hard electric truth. There are no vertical lines on their scales. Only a little digital box connected to the scale by wires. The gauge used to calculate my weight neither fluctuates nor flirts with me as it latches itself onto a final number. I step on the scale and BAM! It spits out a number. A detailed number.

I am no longer a 175 *maybe*. I am a 174.4 definitely. There are no delusions to be had with this number. It is what it is.

I walked into Weight Watchers because my friend, Wendy, walked into Weight Watchers. Weight Watchers, Jenny Craig, the whole lot of weight-loss support groups were not for people like *me*. I'm not *really* fat. I'm not *really* out of control. I know how to lose weight. Let me tell you all about how I lost weight a few years ago. And the few years before that. I don't need some happy, shiny charlatan to smile at me as if I'm a charity case and talk to me about how I just need to follow their program into the Promised Land. I know what I'm doing.

But I have only lost a few pounds since again making the decision I would lose weight. I am not losing more. Something is wrong. Wendy is funny and sharp, one of the most intelligent women I know. If she is finding something here, maybe I can, too. Maybe it's okay.

The Weight Watchers location I choose is the same as Wendy's and a scant distance from where I work. It is the saddest building I have ever stepped foot in. All of the hope has been sucked from this place; empty office fronts dot the hallways inside and you can't help but be struck by the remaining fax machines and copiers no one bothered to remove when the businesses that once occupied these spots shuttered their doors. The only signs of life come from the basement offices containing the weekly neighborhood newspaper, and I have to wonder what they think when they see all of these fat people climbing the stairs toward the Weight Watchers' office. I imagine they are thankful for the obesity epidemic that plagues the country because the droves of overweight Chicagoans paying Weight Watchers $10 a week to attend its meetings keep their rent down.

There is always an obnoxiously long line of people standing outside the entrance, as if they're in line to buy Prince tickets instead of waiting to find out if that cheeseburger they had Wednesday had a lasting effect on their weight-loss efforts. Joining such a public display would be jarring if it weren't for the fact that all of these people are in the same boat you're in and this office is so far removed from reality that you just get in line and wait your turn.

You do this every week. At the same time on the same day. When you begin Weight Watchers, your weigh-in day leaves you feeling like you're a pig being led to the slaughter, your entire day's worth of self-esteem hinging on this week's results. Eventually after adjusting to the program you greet these days with less dread and more pragmatism.

After all, the Weight Watchers POINTS system isn't difficult to figure out. Food is assigned a value in POINTS, based on its ratio of calories, fat, and fiber. All I need to do is use the Weight Watchers slide rule to calculate these three things for a POINTS value. For example, a small pear is worth 1 POINT. I start out each day with 25 POINTS' worth of food that I can eat. I can use those POINTS on twenty-five pears or on a Big Mac and large fry. The choice is mine. I don't need to track four-digit numbers or use spreadsheets to determine if I've eaten more grams of fat than fiber or carbohydrates than protein.

> When you begin Weight Watchers, your weigh-in day leaves you feeling like you're a pig being led to the slaughter, your entire day's worth of self-esteem hinging on this week's results.

I never counted calories or bothered to understand such equations. I like my dietary food values like I like my porn: soft core. The Weight Watchers system is Cinemax for dieters. Meticulous calculations of calories are for those people who like their dieting messy and raw, with extreme close-ups and moaning.

Provided I've stayed within my POINTS range every day for the entire week, I should see some results. There are extra POINTS and activity POINTS and other variables that make all of this work, but I don't pay attention to those things much. My first two months on Weight Watchers find me 12 pounds lighter. I have removed the equivalent of eight medium-sized cantaloupes from my body. I am taught to look at the numbers on the scale the same way I now look at food: simpler.

By New Year's Eve 2002 I've lost three boneless, skinless chicken breasts. A week later, I wind up gaining an entire bucket of chicken, deep-fried and breaded I presume. It takes me the rest of January to lose the fried chicken, and I manage to spend my spring getting serious with my weight-loss efforts. I gain a spoonful of coleslaw every now and then, but mostly I continue to lose more weight from the buffet of fat.

By July 30, 2003, I've lost the cantaloupes, the chicken, as well as a sack of potatoes and eight sticks of butter. According to the woman who tallies my weight that day, I am supposed to be thrilled with the fact that I'm no longer lugging around what amounts to the grocery bag of someone with a penchant for poultry and mild fruit. Mostly I'm just irritated that the weight isn't coming off faster. I want to leave. However, she informs me that I've lost 10 percent of my weight since starting the program and it's a milestone worthy of a key chain. Despite all of my protesting, the meeting leader wants me to come up in front of the group and accept my key chain. I've spent the majority of these meetings sitting in the back of the room, analyzing my weight loss and ignoring the thirty minutes' worth of talk centering around tips, tales, and triumphs regarding the big ugly world of food. The meetings make me feel itchy and stupid.

> I like my dietary food values like I like my porn: soft core.

I relent and agree to stay.

When I walk up to receive my key chain, the thirty-some odd members erupt into applause and cheering. My meeting leader greets me at the front of the room with a hug as if I was the Prodigal Daughter. She hands me my key chain, and I thank her and turn to sit down. I'm stopped.

"Erin, would you share with everyone your secret?" my leader asks me. "How is it that you lost 17.5 pounds and have kept it off?"

I blankly stare at the group. My eyes begin to travel around the room, over the happy, primary-colored posters adorning the walls, all cheerily making mention of weight-loss tips and slogans. I see the hand-made wall hangings bearing cutout feet representing the miles tallied by those taking part in exercise challenges. I see the pictures of local Success Stories and POINTS paraphernalia cluttering the room. All of this hope on display—it reminds me of preschool.

"Because I really believe in Weight Watchers," I respond. "This program is just the best. I'm just the happiest I've ever been."

More applause breaks out and many furiously nod in agreement. I feel like I've just testified and any second now a gospel choir will emerge, the meeting leader will whap me against the forehead chanting Hallelujah's, and I will fall to the ground as a result of my salvation.

I don't know what compelled me to say something so insipid, so contrary to what I was feeling. Maybe it was the summer heat and the fact that there was no ventilation in the room. Maybe it was the sudden swell of encouragement from a group of people who only knew me as the girl who sat through the meetings never saying a word.

Maybe it was just the hope, sprung eternal by the realization that when each of us gets up on the scale every week, there is just as good of a chance that the results will be positive as there is that they will be negative. That it has always been like this.

I get up on the scale the next week. I've only lost a carton of milk. Someone else loses two. I tap her on the shoulder and give her the thumbs-up sign. One woman slumps to her seat, having just been made aware that somewhere along her week's travels she managed to pick up a loaf of bread. She laughs and looks up at me and we exchange conspiratorial smiles.

Still another member loses her first sack of potatoes after weeks of not losing even the slightest morsel; I holler in congratulatory exuberance.

We are all saved. Hallelujah.

The Good, the Bad, and the Neutral (or, Sworn Enemies)

By Robyn Anderson

There exist in my life three different scales: the Bad Scale, the Good Scale, and the Neutral Scale. The Bad Scale lives in my bathroom closet, and it's one of those annoying scales that claims to tell me not only how much I weigh, but also just how much fat I'm hauling around on this ass of mine. It never, *ever* gives me anything approaching a weight I'd be happy to see, and it always gives me a ridiculous number as my fat percentage. One day it tells me I'm 15 percent body fat, and the next day it smirks as it tells me I'm more like 75 percent. I may be pretty clueless when it comes to things like body fat percentage, but I'm *pretty* sure I'm not 75 percent body fat.

I do have one, and only one, good thing to say about the stupid thing, though: When it's decided I weigh a certain number that day, it is rock-solid definite that that's how much I weigh. No matter what I do—run ten miles, cut my hair, drink a gallon of water, carve 10 pounds of fat off my ass with a knife—every time I get on the scale that day it flashes the exact same number at me. I've had to leave the house so I wouldn't lose my mind and toss the scale out the window. Stupid scale. I hate it, but I know it can be trusted—it's like that really annoying friend who has a policy of telling you the truth. You know, the friend to whom you would never pose the question, "Do these spandex shorts make me look fat?" because she would let you know that it actually isn't those spandex shorts that make you look fat. It's your fat that makes you look fat.

The Good Scale lives in my garage. The garage is where I work out every morning, whether it's lifting weights or doing cardio or a combination of the two. We bought the Good Scale years ago when we first started eating right and exercising. It was expensive as hell, can weigh up to 500 pounds, and was better than the cheap scale we had purchased at a discount store years earlier (and then never used). Having the Good Scale in the garage where I'll see it every morning is probably not the best idea. For the most part I pass it by, because weighing myself every day would simply be insanity—some people can handle it, but I end up just driving myself crazy with it.

But sometimes when I'm about to lift weights and looking for a reason to procrastinate, my eye catches the scale and I think, *Hey, I haven't been on the scale in several days!* So I walk over, turn it on, and step on. I call it the Good Scale because it somehow seems to sense when I'm desperate to see a smaller number, and whether I've actually lost any weight it will put its comforting arms around me and show a slightly smaller number. It knows that half a pound is half a pound and it's better than seeing that same damn number or even, heaven forbid, a higher number. I've also learned that if I lean forward *juuuuust* a little, the number will go a tad lower than it was. While you and I know that's not a true weight, not one I can write in the weight-loss chart, sometimes I just need to see the number go a little lower, real or not. The Good Scale is nice, but is also not to be trusted. It's like the friend who tells you that you look wonderful in those spandex shorts despite the look of horror on her face.

It actually isn't those spandex shorts that make you look fat. It's your fat that makes you look fat.

The Neutral Scale lives in the hallway at my doctor's office, and I don't really care what it has to say. I step on the Neutral Scale when I visit my doctor for whatever reason, and that tends to be in the middle of the day when I've eaten breakfast and possibly lunch. I've been drinking water all day long, and I'm fully dressed. Hell, I even wear *shoes* when I step on the scale. The Neutral Scale tells me the truth as of the moment I step on it, but hell, you can't go by *that* number. I mean, fully dressed. Come on. What kind of crazy person believes the number of a scale they've stepped on when fully dressed? You've got to do a little math when you're wearing clothes. That's an established fact, right up there with *the earth is round* and *eating chocolate during your period doesn't count.*

How much does my shirt weigh? Two pounds? And then maybe another 2 for the pants, and the shoes . . . well, those are heavy shoes. Give it 5. So, 2 plus 2, plus 5. My lunch was pretty heavy. Sushi's heavy, right? And then a Diet Coke and yogurt. Let's subtract, oh, 15 pounds. Wait. What did the scale say again? The Neutral Scale isn't really even a friend—it's a passing stranger on the street who can give you her opinion, but who really cares what she thinks? Besides, they never calibrate the scales at doctor's offices anyway. Everyone knows that.

I don't know why the number on any of those stupid scales matters so much to me. I mean, how many times in my life have I woken up feeling absolutely incredible, popped in my contacts, and thought, *Hey, I feel really THIN. I should weigh myself!* only to step on the scale and have my good mood evaporate into the air? A hundred million times, that's how many. It makes *no* sense that in one moment I feel like I've got the world by the tail and the next I feel like my tail is the size of the world. That's an awful lot of power to give a stupid electronic device, and I know that and *you* know that, but still I let the fucking thing rule me.

If I step on the scale and it gives me one number, then I realize there's a wadded-up piece of paper under the scale making it off-balance, and I move the paper and step on the scale again to see a smaller number, how on earth does that make any sense? I didn't actually *lose* weight in the ten seconds it took me to move the paper, so why do I feel like I did? If one scale gives me one number and another a higher number within the same minute, *I still weigh the exact same* both times. So why does my heart sink when I see the higher number?

If I could adequately answer that question, I could no doubt rule the world.

I know I'm not the only one in the world with a particular weighing ritual. Currently I weigh myself on Friday mornings, though I've been known to step on the scale in between from time to time. (But when I step on the scale in between and don't like the number I see, I can comfort myself with the knowledge that I didn't do my weighing ritual and thus the number I see isn't a "true" number. Am I a freak? Why, yes. Yes, I am. But don't even act like you don't have your own weighing ritual, because that would make you even more of a freak than I am.) On Friday mornings I wake up, go to the bathroom, making sure that when I'm done peeing I lean forward to squeeze those last few drops from my bladder. Then I do some morning chores—clean the litter box, do some laundry—while waiting to see if I'll need to pee again.

When I've decided it's time to weigh, I take off every piece of clothing I'm wearing. It's silly to weigh yourself with clothes on (unless, of course, you're at the gym or any other public place), because you can't control whether your clothes have lost weight or not; if they feel they need to lose weight, they're on their own. Weighing yourself with clothes on is like those height and weight charts that say at the bottom, in very small print, *height while wearing two-inch heels.* If you're wearing two-inch heels while you're measuring your height, you need to subtract two inches. Just because you're wearing heels doesn't mean you're *actually* that tall.

But I digress.

Once I'm naked, I pull the scale out of the bathroom closet and turn it on. Then I check myself to be sure I haven't absentmindedly tossed a wet towel or cat over my shoulder. I check to be sure I don't have to pee again. I check to be sure I didn't sweat in my sleep, because if I did and my hair is even slightly damp, I'll blow-dry it. (Sadly, I'm not kidding.) I step on the scale and stare straight ahead, counting to ten. Then I step off the scale and look down to see what the Bad Scale claims I weigh. I weigh myself twice more, because although Bad Scale is always rock-solid and gives me the same number repeatedly, it can't hurt to triple-check.

I usually end my ritual by calling the scale a bad name.

Once the official number is affixed in my mind, I put on my workout clothes and go downstairs where I sit in front of the computer and put off exercising as long as I possibly can. When I do get into the garage on Friday mornings, I inevitably end up on the Good Scale. I don't bother to get undressed, though—that's how little I respect the number Good Scale gives me. I step on Good Scale several times, and sometimes when it's been cold in the garage, Good Scale will give me a number half a pound lower each time I step on it. And you'd better believe I keep stepping on that scale, even if I know the number can't be trusted.

And I usually end this part of the weigh-in ritual by telling Good Scale that it's a good, *good* scale. Because it is. It's not trustworthy, but sometimes a gal needs to be lied to.

I've never really been one to join gyms. I spent time at a gym for women when I was fourteen or so. It was comprised of a single large room with mostly cardio equipment, and I'd do a half-assed workout, most of the time not even working up a sweat before I'd change back into my street clothes and head downstairs to the drugstore where I would—naturally—load up on junk food. When I was nineteen, I had a job on a Navy base and friends who also worked on the base. My friend Liz decided to start working out at the base gym, and the rest of us joined her.

I weighed 200 pounds at the time, so you can imagine how intimidating it was to walk into a gymful of Navy and Marine men and women in amazing shape. I chose to hide my body in oversized sweatpants and T-shirts. Liz met with a trainer who gave her a list of exercises to try, and she in turn showed them to me. Like when I was younger, I'd mostly fool around, trying out different machines and sometimes even sweating a tiny bit, while waiting for her to be done working out. My clearest gym-related memory was when I leg-pressed 300 pounds ten times in a row. When I got home, I told my father how much I'd lifted, expecting him to be impressed by my strength. He said, "Of course you can lift 300 pounds, you've been carrying that much around!"

Did I mention that I weighed 200 pounds at the time?

While going to "work out" at the gym was a good opportunity to watch military guys sweat a lot and to hang out with my friends, there wasn't a whole lot of working out going on. I tried all the machines at least once—though the treadmill was the only one that didn't confuse me—and Liz and I did some boxing (which we sucked at) occasionally.

One memorable time we took turns shooting hoops. Liz is really into sports, so she has a clue what she's doing when it comes to things like trying to get a ball to go through a hoop. I do not. Liz, trying to help me out, suggested I toss the ball at the hoop "granny-style"; that is, bending over and holding the ball between my legs, then straightening up and tossing it at the hoop as I stood up. The ball flew through the air and ended up stuck behind the baseboard. We poked at the ball with a stick, but couldn't get it loose. Finally, two (need I say good-looking?) Marines from the other end of the room came and used their basketball to knock our basketball down from where it was stuck.

When they'd gone back to their game, Liz dared me to do it again. I did, and then I did it a third time. That takes skills the ordinary person just doesn't have, my friends. By the third time the Marines at the other end of the room came to get the ball down for us, they'd ceased being impressed.

I guess that when it comes down to it, I'm just too solitary a person to work out in a gym surrounded by people. My husband and I have built a pretty decent little gym in our garage, and while it doesn't have all the amenities you'd find at a big gym, I never have to wipe a stranger's sweat off the weight bench or wait my turn to do the elliptical machine. It's all mine, and it's available to me whether it's eight in the morning or midnight (though, let's be honest—I've never been struck with the overwhelming urge to do preacher curls at midnight).

And you bet your ass I wear spandex shorts.

I've been on a constant diet for the last two decades. I've lost a total of 789 pounds. By all accounts, I should be hanging from a charm bracelet.

—Erma Bombeck

Dust Up
By Lori Ford

I worship the almighty scale, at least when I'm not nonchalantly stepping over it rather than on it. Its truths haunt me, terrify me, and in fair cases, give me credit when due. It is the judge, it is the jury, it's my own little tell-all book. People talk such nonsense about letting your clothing be the judge, marveling at your biceps not a number on the scale. But I have very strong powers of persuasion over myself. It's so easy to convince myself that these pants—*(breathe)* pull, *(breathe)*—still—*(breathe)*—fit. The smaller sizes secretly retire to the back of my closet and I buy clothing with stretchy waists and larger cuts. I easily convince myself that the entire size 14 has changed; I tell you, it has. I'm still a 12, though I can't find one that fits, even though I was an 8 just last year. It's a myriad of tiny little talks with myself that lead me this way blindly, in certain denial of my true size.

The scale, however, causes me to suck all the air from the bathroom and mutter cusswords I won't even say when I stub my toe. I hate the scale. The scale is against me. I must destroy the scale or at least ignore it, though I will dust it, and don my stretchy pants and casually forget about my baby tees. Size Extra Large, my old friend, makes a newfound presence in the front of my closet and I tout my period as the reason my pants are getting oddly tight (though they'll still be tight next week).

I remember how it used to be, the scale and me, and I miss it. I used to mark my weight daily on a calendar, filling the entire square with the number. Every week I would notate my pounds lost and make adjustments to my diet accordingly. Some weeks I'd maintain and add more exercise or cut out snacks, and some weeks I'd lose 3 pounds and think I was living in my own personal carnival. I considered 1 or 2 pounds good, like getting a B in school. I'd give myself an approving nod as I notated the number below Saturday's weigh-in. At the end of the month, I'd do a monthly wrap-up, and though I was usually disappointed with the number (a month is a long time), I could see the culmination of my efforts and it was amazing. Ah, how I miss the powerful in-control feelings of those days.

The other piece of equipment that's become the dustable object du jour in my house is the treadmill. Originally I begged my mother to purchase it for me as a pre-Christmas gift. I got it home to my apartment and began the frustrating, torturous task of putting it together. After breaking a sweat and blushing with furry, I got it assembled. I plugged it into the wall in the living room, got on, walked for about twenty seconds, got off, unplugged it, moved it into my bedroom, and ignored it for six months.

I dieted for a good solid month until my weight stalled and, pissed at the world that I was reduced to intentional sweating, I pulled the treadmill out from the wall of my bedroom and added it to my schedule four to six days a week for the next six months. I was never a fan, but I did it like a duty, like cleaning the toilet, every day. Not my favorite thing. And it required a bit of serious tunnel vision. There's loads of preparation for getting on the treadmill. I had a whole check list: use the bathroom, put on jogging bra, put on socks and shoes, grab water bottle, shoo kitties out of bedroom (often taunting them out with ribbons), shut the door, put on ceiling fan, put on headphones, turn on television. If any bit of delayed distraction occurred during this time—like a phone call or the kitties giving me a "how can you leave us" look—it was likely I'd skip the day. Once I was on the treadmill it was fine; I just had to make it there. I'd walk in the door after work and go straight into my checklist. I didn't look left or right; I'd just get on the treadmill and go go go until it was done.

Distraction is key. Sometimes a show can distract me from my gerbil race and I can lose myself in the show and my half-hour will be up in record time. Sometimes the perfect music can find me going past my half-hour or dancing around as I put up the treadmill. Sometimes my music seems dull and uninspiring, and the television feels like commercials with short show messages, and time stands still while I continue putting one step in front of another. Those days are the worst.

I've tried every sort of exercise, as I've tried every sort of diet. I once joined a gym to march on my treadmill with other ladies more fit and faster than me. I gripped the handlebars with the terror of falling while strolling as they ran mountain programs on their treadmill without breaking a sweat. Once the gym was crowded and I was forced to wait to use the treadmill, like waiting in line to torture myself, I stopped going, touting that the lines were too long.

I've tried walking around the neighborhood, but it's weather permitting and soon it's too hot, too cold, too windy, too rainy, too sunny, too everything to be bothered to go.

And once I near my goal, exercise is the first to go. I should know by now that exercise must remain part of my program in order to maintain my new lifestyle, but I'll soon come across some modern marvel of science, a skinny girl who doesn't exercise, and I'll convince myself I don't have to do it either. But believing that myth only gets me so far. The truth is, I can only persuade myself into my size XL pants for so many days before I'm out of excuses and out of clothes. I know that in order to stay healthy, and in order to keep those XLs in the back of my closet, I need to stick to my exercise routine. A half-hour a day. It's not that much. There's no reason to put it off. I know that if there's anything I should put off, it's the dusting.

The Magic Number
By Monique van den Berg

There's always a magic number. And you step on the scale—or break out the tape measure, or wriggle into the jeans—hoping to achieve it.

My entire weight-loss career has been a series of magic numbers. Five pounds, 10 pounds, 15 pounds lost. The first 10 percent for which I got a key chain. Twenty-five pounds, 30 pounds, 50 pounds. Size 20 . . . size 16 . . . size 12. Under 250, or 220, or 200. Or the magical 209 pounds, when my BMI officially changes from "obese" to "overweight." Goal weight. Halfway to goal. Total weight lost. Numbers *ad infinitum*.

The magic numbers are useful. They measure both the numerical and some of the non-numerical (fitting into once-tight pants) rewards. Striving for those numbers keeps you accountable, and weighing and measuring yourself keeps you accountable, too.

But numbers aren't everything.

I have clothes in a vast array of sizes. Size XL shirts that are too tight, and L shirts that are too big. Jeans ranging from size 14 to (ugh) size 18. (I refuse to buy size 20 pants ever again, and I don't care if they "run small.") I weigh 5 pounds more at night than I do during the day. I weigh 5 pounds more if I have popcorn at the movies, or take certain drugs, or am having a certain time of the month.

The capricious nature of these numbers is something to keep in mind when you step on the scale—but it shouldn't frighten you away from it entirely. Because the numbers are not, after all, completely meaningless. They can be somewhat arbitrary and somewhat unforgiving and some-what unkind, but they do mean *something*. Which is why right now, I'm afraid to look at them.

After losing 50 pounds, I have a pretty damn good idea of what's going on with my body. And I know I've been eating too much, and moving too little, and I know my weight has been creeping back up. No matter what number the scale says, I know that my jeans should not be size 18. I know that I've been thinner than this. I know that I've paid the price for being unprepared and weak and going out for many fabulous high-calorie meals.

> Numbers aren't everything. . . . I weigh 5 pounds more at night than I do during the day. I weigh 5 pounds more if I have popcorn at the movies, or take certain drugs, or am having a certain time of the month.

I've been on a plan, you see—the plan of self-sabotage. The plan of falling back into old, destructive patterns. The plan that got me here in the first place! And it goes in tiresome, predictable cycles. And three phases.

Here's phase one. I decide I'm beautiful just the way I am (which is true) and everybody loves me (which might also be true) so I should embrace whatever my body wants at that moment (slightly less true) and go eat a dozen Krispy Kremes immediately (not true at all).

This is when I say, "But I am a beautiful person anyway! I am hot stuff! I am so sexy!" and try to paper the walls of my mind with fat-positive slogans—slogans that I do truly believe in, which makes it all the more insidious.

The problem is that in spite of my beauty and my self-confidence, there is a certain weight that I am not comfortable with anymore. For myself. And although I can still think of myself as a beautiful person, if I get outside my comfort zone, I start to feel itchy in my own skin.

My clothes (the tight clothes that show off my curves) are now too tight, clinging to not curves, but *rolls*. And suddenly I am not sexy anymore. Suddenly I can't figure out what to put on that will make me feel the least bit good about myself. If I put on clothes that are too small,

I feel like I am putting my weakness (read: fat) on display. And if I put on clothes that are too big, I feel frumpy and awful.

Worse yet, since I am already "so fat" I give myself a license to go out and eat everything and anything that I'm craving: a package of Oreos, a burger and a milkshake and fries, hot chocolate chip cookies—everything that tastes so good but is such a very bad idea and makes me feel (physically but mostly mentally) like shit as soon as I've finished wolfing it down.

So there's phase one: the sabotage disguised as good self-esteem. Then we move on to phase two: rebellion.

Other people can splurge on McDonald's, so I should be able to, too. Look at that tiny person eating a brownie with hot fudge. It's not fair! Nobody can tell me what to eat! (Mommy issues, mommy issues . . .) I want it so much. I need the carbs/starch/protein/sugar. Why can't I have it?

Of course, I *can,* in moderation. But I've come to realize that my problem is like that of an alcoholic who can't have a sip of wine, because it's a trigger. I'm bad at moderation. Once I eat the McDonald's, I feel like I've "blown it." And since I've already blown it, I might as well have a slice of cheesecake for dessert. And wow, now I've *really* blown it.

And the scale becomes my enemy again. I know I'm going to pay. I know the magic numbers are winding back, back, back in time. I know the direction I'm headed, and I feel ugly, and I feel ashamed, and I feel like pulling on a baggy sweatshirt and eating a pint of Ben & Jerry's. Eating it as quickly and as mindlessly as possible, to hide my shame. Not thinking about it too much, until it's all gone, until it's too late. Not realizing that I didn't even enjoy it. A binge.

Then comes phase three. This is when all food becomes my enemy, and when the ideal for me is not to eat at all. I skip breakfast, I skip dinner, and I eat as little as possible. And then I'm tired, hungry, headachy, unhealthy, and cranky and the whole cycle starts all over again once I've lost (or failed to lose) that 1 or 2 pounds. Because aren't I just beautiful the way I am anyway? And pass the hot fudge!

I don't know at what point—I think it's in phase three—that I decide to go back to what works for me: I surround myself with healthy foods that I like to eat and give myself permission to enjoy those foods. I stop beating myself up over having to "relose" the 5 pounds that I gained in phases one and two. I work to make the scale my friend again.

But I know that it would be easy to regain those 50 pounds. It would be so incredibly easy. All I have to do is give up. All I have to do is stop trying. Put the scale away. Pretend it doesn't matter to me.

One of those irritating-but-true weight-loss slogans is "You can only start from where you are." And every morning I have to wake up and decide to start again, from where I am. I have to decide to keep going. To never give up and never surrender and always, always try again. To forgive myself when, inevitably, I stumble.

And no matter what the scale shows, and no matter what size pants I'm putting on in the morning, that's the real battle that I'm faced with. Because the numbers are a smoke screen. I'm not struggling with the scale, or the tape measure, or the jeans—not really. I'm struggling with myself.

> . . . it would be easy to regain those 50 pounds. It would be so incredibly easy. All I have to do is give up.

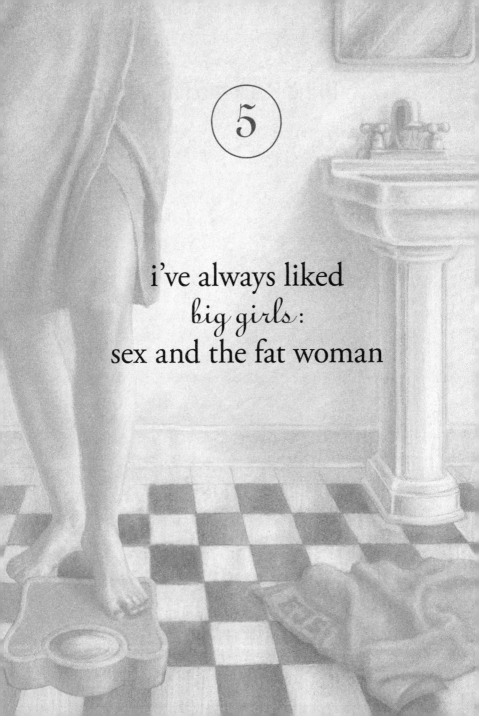

5

i've always liked
big girls:
sex and the fat woman

Bring Back the Fat!

People who have an unhealthy relationship with food are often reminded that food is not love. They have come to believe that food will comfort them, make them stronger. I have never felt this way. I've just always loved fat people.

Each of my grandparents wore clothing of a two-digit size, starting with a 4. We're not talking about a size 16 at the Fashion Bug. I'm talking about Gram's size 44 tents in every flower print available or Pop's size 42 pants that two or three of his granddaughters could have stood in.

My earliest memories are of Gram splitting a bag of M&Ms between my sister and me. While my sister and I somehow maintained our average-girl size, my grandparents stayed big and I loved them for it. Big laps to sit on. Big hands to hold. Big soft shoulders to lean on.

I never realized how much that bigness comforted me until Michelle, my partner of five years, started losing weight. When Michelle decided to lose weight in January 2002, prior to our Commitment Ceremony, I was her biggest cheerleader and lost weight alongside her. We looked great as we exchanged rings that April. After the ceremony, my weight loss petered out. After a summer hiatus, Michelle started counting POINTS again and doing Pilates. She became happier with her body.

By Christina Santos

And then there was me.

"You feel different," I'd say.

"Who is this skinny girl and what did you do with my honey?"

My running commentary may have been my way of trying to adjust to Michelle's new body, but I was driving her crazy. "Shut up, Chris" was Michelle's reply while she giggled and closed her eyes trying to pretend that no one, not even I, could see the new body.

Having my partner lose 90 pounds over the past three years has meant I have had to make adjustments. I have gotten used to the people who look at this tall, thin, freckled girl when we walk down the street. I have even gotten used to 2% milk and part-skim mozzarella cheese.

What I have not gotten used to is that Michelle weighs 90 pounds less. I liked those 90 pounds. I know they weren't healthy. I know they would probably eventually have meant diabetes, heart disease, and joint pain. But those 90 pounds gave me a soft place to lay my head, reassurance when a heavy leg rested on top of mine in bed, and lots of skin to kiss.

I miss the fat. Sometimes the voice in my head screams, "Bring back the fat!" I'm getting used to Michelle's healthier, leaner, body. I am proud of her. But I miss the fat. I guess I'll get used to it.

My Pal Angus
By Julie Ridl

*I*t happened on the bus back from Galway. The bus system in Ireland is fabulous. Big, beautiful, comfortable coaches running the labyrinthine roads that snake all over the island, through narrow aisles of ancient stone walls overgrown with wild roses, negotiating hairpin turns at breathtaking speed. I relied on them because I never knew where I was going and couldn't trust myself to drive in that country. The buses are well used, and on one overfilled bus back from Galway, a man hit on me. We'll call him Angus, naming him after the Irish love god.

Now, when I was a young girl, I enjoyed a reasonable degree of beauty. I was attended to by men and women, not always receiving the type of attention I enjoyed, and sometimes more than I could stand. That is, in the days before anybody named "sexual harassment" or trained anyone not to do it, it was a jungle out there. And I was a jumpy bit of soft flesh, backed against tree after tree until I grew claws and fangs. But a few years as a cocktail waitress left me fairly nimble at putting down unwanted advances.

I don't think I grew my fat as a defense, but these past few decades, the "heavy years," have been blissfully peaceful and put me far out of practice. My skills at rebuff have atrophied. Well, naturally enough: No one ever made a pass at my 252-pound self. No one has made a pass in at least twenty years. Happily married all that time, I haven't needed it or missed it.

Today, I travel more, because travel is more comfortable. I get around more easily; I fit into more places. And I am no longer invisible. Fat women are invisible, sort of. That is, we don't really exist. We do take up space, but we don't exist on a level that requires actual interaction with other people. And particularly not men. I got used to that when I was fat, didn't mind it at all, and really hadn't gotten used to the visibility weight loss gave me when I boarded that bus.

But along comes old Angus. Angus found me in the line for the Ballyvaughan bus outside of Galway station. It was Angus, me, an elderly nun, and an eighty-something-year-old lady loaded down with shopping bags. I guess I looked pretty good in that lineup.

As we boarded the already crowded coach, Angus grabbed the seat next to mine and proceeded to help me untie my jacket from around my waist. He patted my knee, made sure I was comfortable, introduced himself, and made some jokes about not falling asleep, lest I wind up in Lisdoonvarna by mistake. There is apparently a story circulating about a couple of city boys from Dublin falling asleep on the bus and winding up at the end of the line in Lisdoonvarna. I suppose you have to be from Ballyvaughan to get it, but it's so funny to Angus, he can hardly tell it for giggling. He falls into me, across my breasts. It's that funny, this joke.

I'm used to the warmth and friendliness, the arch hospitality of Irish people. They look you in the eye, size you up, and if you are found to be a reasonable sort of Yank, they'll do everything they can to make sure you don't kill yourself by looking the wrong way before crossing the street. Makes me proud of my roots.

But Angus's hospitality quickly oozed over the top. I want to be kind here. Angus was not the sharpest arrow in the quiver. He's an enthusiastic man, who clearly fretted enough through his day about making the right sort of impression that he'd ground his teeth down to nubs. He spent enough time in pubs that if you squeezed him hard, he'd drip hops' oil. Upon discovering that I'm an American, he decided to give me a lesson in Euro coinage. This play allowed him to reach over and over again into the long, long pockets of his green workpants, rubbing his knuckles the entire length of my thigh to retrieve one coin at a time, show it to me, put it back, find the next. Here is a one Euro coin. Here is a penny. Etc. He had lots of change.

He did work hard to impress a girl. Good with his jokes. He punctuated every joke's punch line with a healthy and hot squeeze of my knee, a grab of my hand, and a boozy, breathy, laugh. Did I get it? Did I get it, dear? I was packed as tightly as I could be against the window of my window seat, my backpack on my lap, blocking his squeezes from traveling any farther up my leg, the luxurious coach seats blocking the view of any available empty seats around me.

I was truly flummoxed. I could have yelled at Angus. Could have told him nice guys do not squeeze the knees or rub the thighs of strangers. There are a million things I could have said, I now realize, as I think of them. But I was tired from a day of hiking around Galway, concerned about making an Ugly American scene, and very, very surprised. I completely forgot how to handle even simple, elderly guys like Angus. I dully considered my options, but decided to wait it out.

> Apparently I've still got it, or enough of it to make life as a girl dangerous again.

Not even his several offers to hop off the bus with me to visit one of the many pubs in the many little villages along the road home really pissed me off. My feminist training seemed completely beside the point in this situation. He didn't seem concerned about his sexist assumptions. He wasn't put off by news of my twenty-year marriage. This simply brought a new line of jokes about old married couples, complete with punch-line knee massages.

In one half-hour's time, we reached Angus's stop. One more invitation to join him, and one more decline. He kissed my hand and hopped off the bus, giving me room to breathe and consider the event.

My knee and my face burned for the whole of the next hour while I sat, embarrassed that I hadn't handled this well at all, and stuck with the scents of sweat and alcohol on my skin and in my hair. Angus the Irish love god made me feel like an awkward girl again, a vulnerable object of elderly desire. I forgot how to protect myself, how to see it coming, how to duck. I felt thirteen. I felt twelve. I am shocked and angry with myself for letting my guard down, or for having no guard. For being guardless. There is so much I've forgotten about being a girl. There is so much about being a girl I never wanted back. I have no need or desire for mating skills or displays. I have no desire to redevelop guardedness. I miss my invisibility. I don't want to regrow claws. I actually feel kind-of cheated to be part of a game I don't want to play. I'm the absentminded outfielder who gets hit in the head with the baseball while she's staring at the clouds. Startled. Annoyed. Fully embarrassed. Terribly silly.

On the one hand, how irrelevant, right? On the other hand, apparently I've still got it, or enough of it to make life as a girl dangerous again. Oh, joy. Oh, rapture.

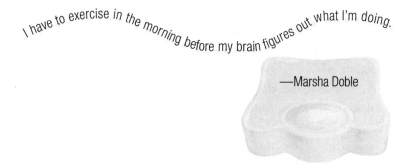

I have to exercise in the morning before my brain figures out what I'm doing.

—Marsha Doble

Dude, Where's My Chest?
By Heather Lockwood

One of the things they never tell you about losing weight is that you may lose your boobs in the process. I'm serious. It happened to me and I'm only thirty-two years old. I still consider myself a young woman. I have yet to conceive any children (no nursing from these mammary glands). Yet, my boobs have become as flat as pancakes. Don't even get me started on sagginess. It is simply not fair. This isn't supposed to be what happens to someone who is in the best shape of her life. I have the best ass I have ever had. My biceps are downright cool. My calves have definition that would rival any pop star's. Yet, my boobs? They are in sad, sad shape.

I didn't notice the changes right away. I was too enamored with the weight loss. Now I'm starting to think it was a distraction tactic used by the leaders of Weight Watchers. The ultimate bait and switch, or "lose" and "lose" as the case may be. Focus on the good stuff and you'll never notice what you are losing in the process.

But then one afternoon while I was trying on clothing at Target in an effort to replace my wardrobe piece by piece, I noticed that the twins were just kind of hanging there in a way I'd never noticed. There was extra room in my bra that my breasts were no longer filling. In response to this, my first thought was, "Great! Now I need to replace my bras, too." But upon closer inspection, I noticed even more than simple weight loss in the chest area. The breasts I've had since puberty had changed drastically. They were no longer perky (not that I ever really used that word to describe them). Instead of fullness, the breasts in the mirror were just sort of flat and hanging there. They had stretch marks. And even though they were obviously smaller than they had been before due to my weight loss, their length was the same. Suddenly the effect reminded me of a pair of empty socks. I had flat, saggy boobs. And with that, I no longer wanted to try on the clothing I'd brought with me into the changing room.

Since this revelation, I've become a bit obsessed. I've been staring at other women's breasts. I've been questioning my coworkers. Many of them have similar stories to tell, only their shrunken breasts came from children and nursing. In essence, they traded in something and got something out of it

> My biceps are downright cool. My calves have definition that would rival any pop star's. Yet, my boobs? They are in sad, sad shape.

that was better. Sure, they lost their breasts, but they had happy, healthy children to show for it. Me? I just lost some weight and now suddenly, I look like I've milked an orphanage.

Until now, I've never paid all that much attention to my boobs. I've never considered myself a highly sexual person and my boobs were just another part of my body. I was never one of those girls in push-up bras and low-cut blouses. I never felt the need to show off my assets or display my sexuality. In fact, while I was at my highest weight, I did my best to hide my breasts just like I hid every other part of my body. My bra collection consisted of tight-fitting contraptions that did their best to constrain and minimize my fullness. On top of the bras, I layered myself in baggy shirts and baggy sweaters. Wispy, floating empire waist dresses were my choice for more formal affairs. I wore them with the firm belief that all shape and form were well hidden from the public view.

Yet, now, I am obsessed. My 36C breasts have deflated to 34Bs and I think about them constantly. I mourn the passing of their former, plumper selves and I wonder what the future will hold. If they handled a 30-pound weight loss so poorly, what will ever happen to them if called upon to nurse? And worse than that, how much more will they sink considering my current young age of thirty-two? In all honestly, I don't have high hopes.

I was reading an article in *Health* magazine the other day that highlighted women and their breasts. Six brave women bared it all on the pages and talked about their feelings regarding this highly feminine area of the body. One woman had recently undergone extensive reconstruction after losing weight herself. She wanted to plump her gals back up. Another woman had had a breast reduction after years of backaches and other health-related challenges due in part to the size of her breasts. Finally, there was a woman who'd had two mastectomies and was left completely breastless. She said that while she missed the breasts she once had, she didn't like using prostheses, either. She was thankful for her health and said if being breast-free got her there, then that was that. Reading this article made me realize how, for women, so much of our femininity, sexuality, and identity is wrapped up in our breasts which, in part, explains my obsession with my suddenly vanishing chest.

There is an ultimate irony in this experience. Now that I'm finally losing weight, I finally want to show off parts of my body that have been hidden for years. I have a renewed confidence and appreciation for a body that I have both abused and cherished for my thirty-two years of life. Yet, I am also ashamed and disappointed to discover a loss that is only in part physical.

Thinking back on it, these feelings are not so different from when I was a teenager. Having your body change is never easy. Then, the issue was waiting for my boobs to arrive in the first place. I remember staying up late watching contraband cable movies. Of them, *Porky's* was my favorite. The shower scene in *Porky's* revealed young women with beautiful, perfect breasts. I mentally compared what I had to these onscreen sirens and literally came up short. In fact, I spent many years waiting for the *Porky's* boobs to magically appear on my body.

But they never did. Sure, I got breasts, but I didn't get *Porky's* breasts. Instead, I got an imperfect set which is probably not so different from the imperfect sets on most women. But I was disappointed nonetheless. My cup to nipple ratio was definitely off. There was never the fullness that I'd seen onscreen. And I certainly wasn't big. But at least I'd developed. That was the important thing. And sometime between the end of high school and beginning of college, I accepted the lot that I was given. In fact, I embraced it. As I came into myself as an adult, I learned to be comfortable with my sexuality. I learned that my boobs were not just an accessory. They were a source of pleasure as well. And until recently, not much further thought went into these gals in the years following that revelation—except, of course, when called upon for duty in the bedroom or when I needed a new bra.

> I think Weight Watchers should have given me some sort of disclaimer, something along the lines of, "Warning: This program may cause shrinkage in all body parts, including those you may still like just as they are."

Yet, here I am now sneaking glances at my chest whenever the opportunity presents itself. I spend enormous amounts of time obsessing about what I have and have not. I also worry and wonder what form the end product will become. Most of all, I am frustrated that this process can't be seamless and easy. Isn't it enough that I've had to eat fewer calories and exercise? Why must I sacrifice my boobs, too?

The rational side of me knows this initial anger and disappointment is really unfounded and unfair. But the emotional side of me can't rationalize that when faced with my reflection in the mirror. I know I will have to come to terms with this new state of being. I just don't know how.

Someone should have warned me. Weight Watchers should have given me some sort of disclaimer, something along the lines of, "Warning: This program may cause shrinkage in all body parts, including those you may still like just as they are." I didn't see this coming and I'm reeling from the effects, not to mention spending a fair amount of cash on the first pushup bras I've ever purchased in my life.

What I need to realize is that change is inevitable. I need to understand that I am still a work in progress, even at age thirty-two. And, like those women in the magazine, I need to be proud of my breasts, as flat and squishy as they may be. They are a symbol of my womanhood. They are a source of pleasure. They are part of this body that I know and love. So what if they have stretch marks now? At the end of the day, they tell a lot of stories, and I wouldn't be the same woman without them.

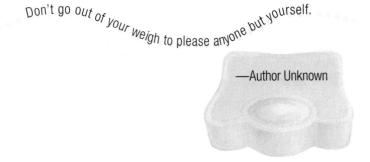

Don't go out of your weigh to please anyone but yourself.

—Author Unknown

The Vagina Returns
By Shauna Marsh

"So, how's *the Body* looking these days?"

My mother had called up for her weekly Status Report. Since I moved from Australia to Britain, she's had to rely on phone calls, instead of just dropping by to see if my pants have fallen down yet.

"Oh, it's looking all right!"

"So do you feel good about yourself?"

"Indeed I do."

"So do you feel . . . sexy?"

"What?"

"I *said,* do . . . you . . . feel . . . sexy?"

"I'm not going to talk about that with you!"

"*Aww, c'mon,* why not?" she insisted. "I was sexy once, you know!"

I quickly changed the subject, but her question haunted me. Did I feel sexy? Had I *ever* felt sexy?

When I weighed 350 pounds, I was so consumed with self-loathing that I felt I didn't have the right to consider myself sexy. I knew many overweight women had active sex lives with boys chasing them all over the town, but I didn't want any of that. The thought of unveiling acres of pale, wobbling flesh to a lover made me feel ill. I'd had a few relationships, but for the most part I did my best to avoid them. I felt safer being invisible to the opposite sex.

Still, I was full of longings and desires like any red-blooded woman. I had a wild and active sex life, but it all took place in my head. It was a steamy ménage à trois—me, my imagination, and a buzzing friend called Mr. Shakey. Lying in the dark with the gentle hum of two AA batteries, my weight wasn't an issue. I could be anyone I wanted to be, be with anyone I wanted. I was safe from criticism and rejection . . . and I could bend like a pretzel.

Things slowly changed when I began los-ing weight. I started to like my body, even though I was still obese. My weight-loss jour-ney was going to take a long time, so I realized

> I had a wild and active sex life, but it all took place in my head.

there was no sense waiting for some miniscule dress size to be kind to myself. I began to appreciate my curves, the beginnings of a waist and shapely shoulders.

I had a wondrous moment one morning as I got out of the shower. Looking in the mirror, I was startled by the sight of a bright red *thing* between my legs.

What the hell?

It was my pubic hair! And gosh darn it, *a vagina!* My girly bits were back, previously obscured by the tsunami of flesh that was my stomach. It was a visual reminder that I was indeed a hot young mama.

I began to consider the idea that maybe I was just a little bit sexy.

But then, I fell in love.

It was terrifying. Until then, my changing body was a beautiful, pri-vate thing, like an inventor working on a top-secret project in a dingy laboratory. But now someone else had noticed it, and I was going to have to unleash the beast in public.

On the one hand, you had the New Foxy Shauna who wanted to ravage and be ravaged, who wanted it now and in every way possible and twice on Sundays. But there also lurked the Old Shauna, riddled with paranoia and devoid of self-esteem. There was no shortage of desire; I was always mentally undressing the guy—the problem was all in the execution. How do you reconcile the lusty thoughts in your head with the awkwardness of your body? How do you get the confidence to *feel* instead of *think?*

Sometimes I am completely distracted by my body in all its apparent faultiness. There's no stopping the constant mental Director's Commentary during sex:

"You are beautiful," my boyfriend will say.

"Surely you jest," blurts the voice in my head.

Instead of enjoying the moment, I'm in a constant panic over what will happen next and how my lumpy form won't be able to handle it. Shall we try a new position? Oh great, another unflattering way to rearrange my bulk! You want me to go on top? But surely that's my worst possible angle. And why are your eyes closed? Are your eyes closed in ecstasy or are you avoiding the sight of my jiggling boobs? Lord, please let it be ecstasy!

My boyfriend couldn't be any more sweet, loving, and appreciative of my body. I know it's me who needs come to term with the curves. I need to let go so he can cuddle up behind me and run his hand over my body *without* me hurriedly sucking in my stomach.

I used to have a Game Plan. I would lose all my weight and shake off all my body issues, and *then* I would I become a sex goddess and be ready to meet Mr. Right. But of course it doesn't happen that way. Mr. Right doesn't care about an extra 40 pounds. Everyone has bundles of insecurities about their bodies, whether they're fat or thin, and there's no greater showcase for insecurities than sex.

These days I make a conscious effort to relax, to look in the mirror each day and like my body just how it is. If there's any hope of overcoming my old demons, I have to make a conscious decision to change my thinking and not to listen to that voice. Now the Director's Commentary is different: *Girl, just shut up and enjoy the ride!*

So to speak.

Some Guy's Fat Chick
By Erin J. Shea

*H*ad someone wanted to have sex with me in high school, I would have grabbed his hand and dragged his ass to home base faster than you can say, "Is your mom home?"

To all of those boys I knew in high school: You totally missed your chance. I was way easier than all of those girls who just *looked* easy. I wanted to get laid with a capital "Let's Get It On." I wanted to fumble and grope and get hot and sweaty in the dark of some guy's bedroom on a late Saturday afternoon when we were supposed to be studying algebra but were suddenly overcome by the heady intoxication of phrases such as "combining like terms" and forced to combine some terms of our own until his mother started banging on the door to ask "Why is it so quiet in there? You kids want some pizza?"

There was no sex for me. Sex happened for seemingly everyone else around me. My free time was spent writing for the school paper, eating copious amounts of chicken nuggets to pass the time between customers as I manned the drive-thru at Wendy's, and collecting Pearl Jam imports. Chubby and slightly awkward, I got off on discussing politics, eschewed all things feminine, and despite my raging hormones and attempts to unleash them onto unsuspecting boys, I was always the Best Friend.

I felt like a portly round peg among a grid of square holes that would have done anything for some sharper edges. Or maybe just a little less belly fat.

In the face of my lack of dates on Date Night, I was banking that my brand of sexuality would go over big in college, where wire-rimmed, goateed poet boys would find my rants about conformity and feminism a turn-on and whisk me away to their dorm rooms to read Shakespeare by candlelight. And it did—on several occasions. There was Keith, a tall, thin engineering major with fabulous taste in music and dark eyes that danced when he talked about how all he wanted to do was switch his major to philosophy. There was Robert, the charming radio aficionado with a penchant for 1960s' comedians and scooters. I

> I felt like a portly round peg among a grid of square holes that would have done anything for some sharper edges. Or maybe just a little less belly fat.

can't forget Adam, the frat boy who would play Big Head Todd and the Monsters and had a near-encyclopedic memory of every column written by Mike Royko.

I happily dated a gaggle of men who romanced and courted me in a manner I had always dreamed about: nights filled with passionate kissing and walks around the campus quad; days containing long, heated discussions about music and writing. I no longer felt physically unattractive and gave my weight nary a second thought; after all, that many boyfriends couldn't be wrong.

Then I met Jason and everything changed.

I was beginning my senior year of college when we met. Jason understood Nabokov, listened to Ani DiFranco, and didn't own a television set. We would spend hours in cafés not talking, but sipping wine and passing notes to each other across the table. He was passionate and romantic.

I had never felt so beautiful, so confident, and so sexy in my entire life.

One night over Sapphire tonics at a bar, we were having a pleasant conversation about our parents when he dropped the following on me: "My mom is a big woman. I guess that's why I've always liked big girls. Girls like you."

"What do you mean, 'Girls like me'? What the hell is that supposed to mean?" I was livid. In that moment I became both the victim of some guy's oedipal complex *and* a Big Girl to boot. Intellectually I could have handled Freud, but I couldn't wrap my brain around the fact that Jason, who made me feel more beautiful and desired than anyone before him, had a Fat Chick Thing and therefore I was a Fat Chick.

How could I be a Fat Chick? Fat Chicks didn't get guys like this! Fat Chicks didn't date any of the kinds of guys I've dated! Did *they* all have a Fat Chick Thing, too?

I was so angry and hurt I stopped the conversation in its tracks. He started to explain how my rolls of soft flesh were sexy to him, but I wanted none of it. There was no room in my life for a Botticellian self-image, no matter how true it may have been. In my head, fat did not equal sexy.

Jason and I broke up not long after he made this revelation. While Jason's thing for Big Girls did not directly contribute to the end of our relationship, it did impact how I saw myself, and as a result, it affected my behavior. All of my insecurities climbed their way to the surface and I began to question his every move. When he would wrap his arms around my waist, I'd swat him away. Not surprisingly, our love life was as interesting as watching paint dry.

I was so self-conscious. I felt so ugly—so . . . *fat*.

The following summer, immediately after our breakup, I began a diet and fitness routine that included anything made with Olestra, Wild Turkey sours, cigarettes, and three hours of cardio a day. I began to take diet supplements washed down with 64 ounces of Diet Coke. By the time September rolled around, no one recognized me. Not even my own sister. Never before was I so determined to lose weight. Never again would I be some guy's Fat Chick.

I managed to lose 50 pounds in three and a half months and start dating Murray.

Poorly suited for each other from the get-go, Murray and I both had expectations for each other that neither could live up to, least of all me. Predictably, in six months' time I gained back the weight I'd lost, thanks to my need to eat solid foods again and the general sense of malaise I had about my life. The more weight I gained, the angrier I was at Murray for worrying about why it was happening. The loss of my svelte body never upset Murray as much as the loss of the confident, self-assured girl who inhabited it, though that never stopped me from convincing myself, and Murray, that he meant otherwise.

Murray and I broke up within the year. I was fat again and fat did not equal sexy.

Midway through out first date at a bar in the Lincoln Park neighborhood of Chicago, Erik asked me if I was hungry and if I liked Buffalo wings.

I didn't want to be on this date; I had been single for a year since Murray. Restoring my self-image took moving back home to Chicago from my college town of Peoria, Illinois, a new job, time, and some perspective. I wasn't willing to take the chance of ruining a good thing.

"There is a bar on the north side that serves the best Buffalo wings," Erik said. "Would you want to go there? They pour a great Guinness, too."

"Sure," I replied, immediately unsure if moving our date to a new location was wise, especially one that purported to serve the best Buffalo wings in town. If I was smart, I thought, I'd order a grilled chicken salad.

We entered the bar and sat down, carrying on our conversation. Erik entertained me with stories from his childhood—about how he used to put his youngest sister, Stacey, in the middle of the street and douse her in ketchup so he and his brother, Sean, could pretend to be reporters who stumbled upon a murder. The more we talked, the more we learned how much we had in common. He put me at ease and made me laugh.

"What do you think of ordering twenty-four Buffalo wings?" he asked.

"I think I'm going to get a salad, so you can get a smaller order for yourself," I said.

"Salads are no fun! Let's get the Buffalo wings!"

Salads are no fun. The words reverberated through my head like a gong. No fun. I am no fun. For the past two years I had developed an outrageously high standard of beauty that equaled an even higher standard for myself, simply because I didn't want to see myself as a Fat Chick. I had traded in fun for thin, and no matter how much better my self-image was than it had been in the past, I had forgotten that relationships aren't just about sex and the validation of my own sexuality. They were also about having some fun, and in the end, nothing is sexier than a girl who knows how to have some fun.

"Buffalo wings and Guinness it is then," I said.

> I had traded in fun for thin, and no matter how much better my self-image was than it had been in the past, I had forgotten that relationships aren't just about sex and the validation of my own sexuality.

> The chief excitement in a woman's life is spotting women who are fatter than she is.
>
> —Author Unknown

Sexual Healing
By Robyn Anderson

I have sex. I have lots of sex. I have lots of *good* sex. And at this moment, I weigh 243 pounds. Hollywood would have you believe that I spend my time sitting on the couch shoving ice cream in my face instead of in the bedroom having lots of good sex with a man I outweigh by 40 pounds. A man who loves me and wants to have sex with me. Is he a *freak*? I mean, for God's sake, I weigh 243 pounds! And he *wants* to have sex with me, regularly.

Not only is he not a freak, he's also not alone. I've been fat my entire adult life, I look nothing like the heroines in the movies—in fact, I weigh at least twice what most of them do—and yet I've *managed* to have sex with decent guys who respect me and want to continue having sex with me. The fact is that although I've never looked like (*insert the Hollywood goddess of your choice*), I've had boyfriends since I was sixteen. Several of those boyfriends were rake-thin, without an extra ounce of fat on their bodies, but never they made me feel like my body, with plenty of extra ounces of fat, was ever anything other than what they desired.

> I have lots of *good* sex. And at this moment, I weigh 243 pounds.

I once had a boyfriend who was overweight. We dated for several months when I was seventeen, then broke up and got back together a few times. He joined the Navy during one of the times our relationship was back on, and while he was at boot camp sent me a letter suggesting we have a "contest" to see who could lose the most weight while he was gone. Fun! Though he may not have expressly meant "*Damn*, you're fat!"—no doubt he thought he was being subtle—I could read between the lines, and our relationship didn't last much longer.

My first husband was the roommate of my best friend's boyfriend and I would say it's a safe bet that he was attracted to me immediately. We went out for a little while, stopped seeing each other when our mutual friends broke up, and then a few months later when I decided that it was time for me to have sex for the first time, we got back together.

I was nineteen. We had sex in his single bed, in the barracks on the Navy base while his roommates were out. Not the most romantic experience, but I wasn't looking for romance. I was looking for sex.

Five months later we moved into an apartment together. We were young and stupid and not terribly careful, and we had lots and lots of sex. The more sex we had, the more sex I wanted, and the more comfortable I was being naked around him, walking around without a stitch on, even though I'd gained weight since we first got together. He never made me feel uncomfortable about my body in those first few months, despite the fact that I outweighed him by a good 75 pounds.

He liked my body, and I almost did, too.

Six months after we moved in together, we were married and I was pregnant. I took the idea of "eating for two" to heart, and gained 50 pounds during my pregnancy. Those 50 pounds didn't slow down our sex life, though the morning sickness put a damper on it for a while, and he always made it clear that he enjoyed the changes pregnancy brought to my body. I had the baby—suffice it to say she didn't weigh 50 pounds—and in the months that followed as I recovered from a C-section and tried to figure out what that squalling red-faced baby *wanted*, I felt completely uncomfortable in my body. I initially lost some of the weight I'd gained while pregnant, but it wasn't long before I was gaining again.

We had a couple of not-very-satisfactory experiences, and then when our daughter was six months old, *it* happened. Something I would bet he didn't remember the next day, but has stuck with me over the past fifteen years.

We were lying in bed, and I said something derogatory about how fat I'd gotten. He responded with, "Well, I guess you should try to lose weight then, huh?" Whether he was just trying to be helpful in his own way or really meant that my weight was starting to bother him, I don't know. I *do* know that I immediately believed he meant the latter, and in the remaining seven years of our marriage we probably had sex less than twenty times.

Sadly, I can report that when it's been a certain amount of time, maybe a few months, you don't really miss sex. You miss the kissing and touching, the intimacy, but you don't miss the sex act itself all that much. Or maybe I can only speak for myself.

In my current marriage, I find that my husband Fred has little patience for bullshit. Which is to say, when I'm feeling particularly fat and want to keep my shirt on during sex, he won't put up with it. He wants that shirt on the floor with the rest of my clothes. The fact that he wants to see me naked—that when I'm running from the bathroom to the closet to get dressed, he'll peek over his book to catch a sight of my naked ass—that he looks at me naked and feels desire, that goes a long way to heal the trauma of that long-ago "Well, I guess you should try to lose weight then, huh?" from my first husband.

So, yes, we have sex. We have lots of sex, and we've been married for more than five years. We recently went on vacation for three days, and while I wouldn't be so crass as to share actual numbers . . . well, let's just say I'd need more than one hand to count that high. Pretty good for an old married couple pushing forty, wouldn't you say?

Take that, Jennifer Aniston. I'll see your Brad Pitt and raise you one Fred any day.

The Naked Truth
By Lori Ford

I try to pretend like nothing's changed. After all, a woman is never happy with her body, right? He met me when I had lost a lot of weight. I was practically at goal weight. I wore a black strapless dress with a slight A-line flare at the bottom, black kitten heels, and pulled my hair back in a bun (it was raining and my hair threatened to frizz). I felt very pretty. I feel pretty at anything less than 138 pounds. And yet there was the resilient arm flab, skin hanging ever so slightly that made me gape at the new pictures of me—the girl who looks like what I always thought I looked like, except that weird bit of arm skin.

Naked, I was most concerned with my deflated boobs. It seemed cruel that after all the hard work of losing weight my body still wasn't perfect, that I still wasn't happy with it. But my new, less shapely boobs were a small price to pay. It was freeing, my size. I could get up to use the bathroom without wanting to grab something to cover me. I didn't care whether the lights were on or off or what position I was in. When he told me I was beautiful, I felt it for the first time in my life.

But my weight started returning. At first I marveled in my returned cleavage. But mostly I mourned the loss of my naked self-confidence by eating more pizza. The food numbed me from my inadequacy.

Even as I continue to gain, I can't help but think if I were skinny he couldn't resist me. But eating takes me further from the body in which I feel good—the body I feel he needs to see in order to desire me. I know this and yet I continue to eat and eat.

Naked jaunts to the bathroom now have an aura of quickness and hiding rather than my former sexy swagger. His eyes don't follow me like they used to. The sex has waned. When we do have sex, I spend the time thinking about my fat, if it's touching him, if he can tell. Even if my fat hasn't affected him, it's certainly affected me. I'm a wreck. He tells me I'm beautiful every day, often multiple times a day. He tells me in new ways, believable ways, and yet I continue to discount the compliments, his heart, with my every negative thought.

The black strapless dress doesn't fit like it used to. Now when we dress for a nice night out, I'll often break into a frustrating sweat trying to find something that fits me. Pantyhose resist me and trap the fat of my stomach, reminding me I'm a prisoner of my own body. All this should be enough to convince me to diet, to return to my old body. I've never understood why the eventual weight regain comes back with such little fight. Certainly, the power of a brownie isn't worth all this discomfort and mental torture. Certainly, a sexy body is worth more than a deep-dish pizza.

The other day he came home early from work. I was in the bath after a heavy workout session on my treadmill. My body was lumping out of the water like a blurry Loch Ness Monster photo. I screeched the shower curtain closed and tried to cover the panic in my voice. Did he see it? Did it disgust him? Did he flinch when he saw me?

I know a lot of overweight women still feel very sexy and are very sexual. They embrace their curves, ample breasts, flushed faces. They know the men in their lives love them and that makes them feel free. But I'm hypersensitive when I'm overweight. Every nuance must be because I'm fat. If he's not in the mood, it's because I'm fat. If his eyes don't follow me longingly as I leave the bed, it must be because I'm fat. Every day that we don't have sex or we do but with clothing on or lights off, it has to be because I'm fat. And even if it's not because I'm fat, the simple fact that I *think* it is affects my self-confidence and appearance. It's a self-fulfilling prophecy. It drives me crazy. It makes me hungry.

Big Bottom
By Monique van den Berg

Question: "Why is a fat girl like a moped?"

Answer: "They're both fun to ride, until your friends see you."

It's amazing how much one lame attempt at humor can cut to the heart of the matter. This joke exactly confirms my theory about society and sex and Fat Girls.

I think that in a societal vacuum, a lot of guys would prefer a sensual Kate Winslet to a bony Calista Flockhart. Queen Latifah is probably a lot more fun to touch than Lara Flynn Boyle. But society tells men that if they are with a Fat Chick, it is because they "can't do any better." Society makes big women feel shame for being big, and it makes our partners feel ashamed to be with us. Fat women are not trophies, not *Playboy* models, and certainly not sexual beings. It's bullshit, but it's *not* all in our heads.

In the world of media, the fat woman is always portrayed as the sexless next-door neighbor or, worse, the desperate and horny lonely heart. She's the outcast, the loner, the misfit. She's the girl who will never be happy and never find love unless she loses 20 (because she's never really *that* overweight) pounds. This rule is reinforced over and over again, until it becomes so ingrained in our heads that we're permanently screwed up. Fat Girls are not sexy.

The rare exception to this portrayal is something that inspires deep gratitude. I'll never forget watching the curvy girl get the hottest guy in *Hairspray*—or that episode of *Three's Company* when Jack Tripper makes fat Bernice feel sexy. And, uh, I can't think of a third example.

160

Only in the black community is "bigness" celebrated. We aren't fat; we have kickin' curves. We are bootylicious. Men like big butts and they cannot lie. Without the stigma of shame—with, instead, a social code of acceptance—men are free to express their preferences.

I was lucky. These days, meeting someone who proudly expressed a preference for big girls would probably make me feel conflicted. I would wonder about their hidden agendas. I've heard people say that "a Fat Girl will do anything in bed" or that "Fat Girls will try harder to please you" and somehow I have become riddled with strange sexual expectations. Do I have to give head for an hour and a half? Do I have to lie back and moan while he kneads my breasts like dough? Do I have to dress up like Ursula the Sea Witch and slap him around a little? Who knows?

> Do I have to dress up like Ursula the Sea Witch and slap him around a little? Who knows?

At the time, though, when I was eighteen years old and still somewhat unjaded, I took Jake at his word: He just liked curvy chicks. One of my first sexual experiences was an affirming one. This did not, however, mark the end of my self-consciousness. Far from it.

Although I hadn't learned to distrust my sexual body, I was already ashamed of my fat, thanks to all of those adults whose "helpful criticism" fed my burgeoning self-loathing: "You should cut down on the cookies," "You have a nice personality," and the classic "You would be so pretty, if only you lost weight." (If I ever hear any adult say that about any child or any teenager, I might deck them. This sentence should be permanently banned from the English language.)

So I could believe that I was sexy and that Jake wanted me, but the "me" he wanted—I was convinced—was not the jiggly, unsightly girl in the mirror, but the one pressed close to him, the pillowy body that wasn't brittle or bony, but yielding and soft. I understood that he'd want to touch me and hold me and fuck me, but not that he'd want to look at me.

After we had sex the first time, in the middle of the night, I had to use his bathroom. I remember not wanting to get out of bed because if he saw me, I knew he'd never want to touch me again. I longed for a towel to cover myself with as I ran across the room. Grateful that he was still asleep, I got back into bed and pressed my body close to his. I wanted to avoid, at any cost, that arm's-length distance he would need to take a good look at me. And look at myself naked? Never. Not ever.

I've looked at my naked body since then, and I still don't love what I see. I can appreciate my clothed body, and I can appreciate the touchability of my nude form, but I can't imagine myself proudly prancing around in front of my partner as if it could in any way be arousing. I rely on touch, on the way my body feels pressed against his. Sometimes I rely on low-cut shirts. (Big tits: the Fat Chick's ace in the hole.)

> I rely on touch, on the urgency of kisses, on the way my body feels pressed against his.

When I was that relatively innocent eighteen-year-old girl, I had a best friend (also a big girl) who had been sleeping around since she was thirteen. She was so unabashed about it that I actually witnessed it for myself once or twice, not by choice. But one story she told really stuck with me.

One day, she stripped for her boyfriend. She peeled off her clothes item by item, with some music playing, and tossed her underwear over his head, seducing him. And he told her that he thought her striptease was the sexiest thing ever—that her confidence was sexy.

She told me her secret: she didn't feel confident at all! She hated her body. But she thought since she had to get naked anyway, she might as well try and fake it. If she pretended she didn't hate her body, maybe he wouldn't hate it either. And it worked. Her chutzpah made her sexy, and it made her feel like he wanted her, flab and fat rolls and all.

I admired her, but I couldn't emulate her. It's been ten years since I heard that story, and I still haven't stripped for anyone.

I did take a page from her book in terms of confidence, though. I learned that confidence is the single sexiest trait a girl can have. And as a result I've rarely been without boyfriends, prospects, make-out partners, lovers. I'm a flirt, and I'm a catch, and I have fun. My issues have, however, affected my relationships at times.

I know that my last boyfriend thought I was sexy, but I was heavier than I had ever been in my life, and our sex life suffered for it. When I'm not happy with my body, the last thing I want to do is show it off. I'd rather have sex under the covers, with the lights low.

I don't know how much of this is just generic sexual insecurity, as experienced by all women. Margaret Cho had a great response to the article in *Cosmo* about how to look your best during sex: "If you care what I look like when you're fucking me, you shouldn't be fucking me in the first place." But there's a *Cosmo* girl in all of us, threatening to make her grating little voice heard: "Lie on your back so your stomach is flatter." "Don't get on top; it's very unattractive." "Make sure the noises and faces you make are ladylike."

That *Cosmo* girl must be a lousy lay.

One thing that helped me like my sexual body a little better was having sex with women who had shapes similar to mine. The women I find attractive are not thin, and whether that's because I'm threatened by thin women or have a genuine preference for larger ones, I couldn't say. I like the feel of flesh. I like women who look like me; my attraction makes me feel attractive. In my dalliances with women, I am the ultimate egomaniac.

Fifty pounds ago, I was dating a guy who loved my butt. He called it "fabulous" and couldn't stop touching it. He was so blatantly enthusiastic about it that I've never looked at my flabby white ass the same way again. And now I think of myself as a girl with, if not a fabulous ass, at least nothing to be ashamed of.

I guess it is too bad that it takes positive reinforcement from outside ourselves to feel good about ourselves, but, hey: it's sex. Sex taps into our deepest insecurities. It's not only large women who use sex for reinforcement. We all want to be reassured that we're attractive; that's what half of sex is all about. It's a weird kind of social power play that nobody really understands, or at least I don't.

The real shame here is that most guys probably genuinely don't notice the body flaws we agonize over. I was lying in bed with my current partner, complaining about my arm flab, and he said I didn't have any. I insisted that I do (because I *do*) and he said, "I'm right here; we're naked in bed together. It's all in your head." (A guy who doesn't believe in arm flab? Be still my heart.)

I got involved with this guy the same I week I joined Weight Watchers. He found me attractive when I was 40 pounds heavier. And somehow he has managed the magical trick of supporting my efforts and still making me feel sexy at every stage along the way. One week, I thought I'd gained weight, when in fact I'd lost it. And he said, "I knew you would." I asked, "How do you know?" "I've done a lot of appreciation of your body, you know. I'm pretty familiar with it. I can tell when it's changing."

And it doesn't make me feel like he's critical of my body, although I suppose I could take it that way. I focus on the part where he says he's been appreciating my body all along. I focus on the fact that I can lie in bed and let him run his hand up and down the length of my body, even the places that make me most tense, and feel completely relaxed.

Maybe six months or 10 pounds from now I'll finally get up the nerve to strip for him. Because I have a feeling that he'll still be around, appreciating my body. And maybe by that time, I will have learned how to appreciate it too.

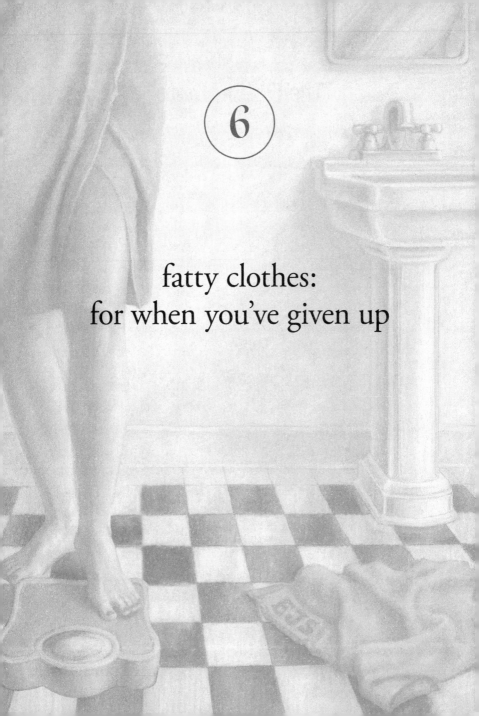

6

fatty clothes:
for when you've given up

The Fat Girl Store

At ten, I dressed, much of the time, like a little old lady.

I can remember a maroon button-down shirt made of gauzy fabric with a crisscross pattern comprised of gold thread. I wore it for my school picture. At your local senior center, I would have been the most well-turned-out woman at the pinochle tournament.

They didn't make normal clothes for little Fat Girls back then. There were T-shirts and there were jeans, but the jeans usually had some particular socially clumsy tell, something that made it clear that the girl wearing them was many things, but certainly not cool. Appliquéd sweatshirts. Polyester stretch pants. No, I'm serious. *Polyester stretch pants.* On a ten-year-old. I suppose the theory was that while skinny little girls wanted to be Madonna, Fat Girls wanted to be Rue McClanahan.

As an adult, sometimes, it's all I can do not to wander the store racks, talking inside my head to the people who made whatever I'm looking at. *No, thank you, that looks too much like my shower curtain. No, thank you, I make it a rule not to wear anything with kitties on it.*

> They say you dress for who you want to be; I suppose the theory was that while skinny little girls wanted to be Madonna, Fat Girls wanted to be Rue McClanahan.

By Linda Holmes

What you wear says something. "I am having a lazy Saturday." "My wife made me wear this." "I had the tomato soup for lunch." Fat Girls are consigned to clothes that seem to say . . . *I would not presume.*

I would not presume to try to look cute. To try to be cool. To spy on myself in the mirror and smile in a way that might seem vain. To suspect that hideous clothes might look ugly because they are ugly, and not because I am. *I would not presume.*

There's a lot of irony buried in my recollections of getting bigger through high school while slowly shrinking in a hundred ways. I lost that ability to presume, and it tied me in knots for years.

How do you do anything of significance if you don't presume? You presume to think you can run a marathon. You presume to think you can lose 50 pounds, or 100, or 200.

A certain measure of vanity is healthy. I don't wear things I hate. I don't buy things that are ugly.

It seems like hyperbole to suggest that those ugly, unfashionable clothes are part of ushering Fat Girls into a lifetime of apologizing for being in the room, but they are. And no, ugly pants in junior high school are not the unique province of the Fat Girl, nor is that probably the biggest problem she has. But I swear, I learned to lower my expectations—to never presume—in dressing rooms at Sears, and it took a long time to unlearn.

What to Wear
By Julie Ridl

After the big weight loss, one of the strangest and most expensive transformations in my life took place in my closet. Obviously, I had to replace all of my clothes as the weight came off.

This freed me from the fat-lady stores. *Halle-freaking-lujah.*

The white-hot hatred I held for those places kept me out of them as much as possible. I shopped only once every two years, and then with great anger and speed. At home, I would prepare for these blitzes by running a tape measure around myself, looking up my probable size on a size chart, and swallowing a Xanax. Then I ran through these stores and pulled things from racks, quickly looking at the seams, then stacking stuff at the cash register, rejecting all help. I never tried anything on. I'd take things home and hope for the best, never returning anything that didn't work. That's how much I hated these places.

Why? Not because they forced me to admit my fatness. Not because I didn't like walking around with the fat-lady-store logo on my shopping bag, although the idea that heavy women needed to be sequestered into other stores bothered the hell out of me.

No. What made me angry was this: the clothes were stupid. Or they were crappily constructed. Usually both. All cloying patterns and off colors, crappy fabrics, sloppy stitching, laces, appliqués, and ruffles that make large women look infantile.

Why would large women want this stuff, exactly? Are our brains structured differently? Do our eyes filter light, form, color, pattern differently than the eyes of average-sized human beings? Do we not watch the same programs, read the same magazines, and so long for the same styles and fabrics? Why are we given something different? I know we're thought to be stupid, but how stupid would we have to be to not know that these clothes are inferior in every way?

We rarely complain, though, because we feel we don't deserve the good stuff.

We know jeans are designed first for the runway, with pockets tooled once for the production line. As sizes grow larger, the pockets and patches remain in the sample size, so that the whole garment looks ridiculous and ill-proportioned once it's sized to fit the majority of the population. I gave up on jeans and patch pockets for years.

Why would large women want clothing from fat-lady stores, exactly? Are our brains structured differently? Do our eyes filter light, form, color, pattern differently than the eyes of average-sized human beings?

Designers' and engineers' preferences for the nontypical small body affect clothing physics. Straps don't stay up on rounded shoulders. Smaller calves determine sock length and performance, so socks never stayed up on me. Forget knee-high boots. Your no-line panty styles? Please. Who cuts these things?

It's been an uncomfortable and annoying life. And while the world is just starting to get more comfortable for the heavy majority—T-style bra straps, stretch-suede boots, gorgeous new clothing lines, thank goodness—I have joined the minority ranks.

It's been fun in part because I get to break the hard-and-fast rules about dressing that I wrote and followed for the past twenty years. I developed my rules to distract those around me, as well as myself, into looking at my face rather than my body:

- Black or other very dark colors below the waist: long black skirts, long black pants, black socks, black shoes (Cover it all.)

- Fabrics in matte, not shiny, to absorb, not reflect, light (Reflected light draws attention to size.)
- No patterns (Big patterns made me look like a psychedelic bus. Small patterns made me look like a giant psychedelic bus.); no plaid
- Fine textures work (Shantung, yes. Crepe was my friend.)
- Shirts needed to flow or hang, never cling
- No shoulder pads
- Solid-color, one-color dressing
- Simple, clean lines
- Long sleeves (until I couldn't take the heat, and then elbow-length sleeves)
- Men's pinpoint cotton dress shirts, sleeves rolled for summer (Big enough, well-made, and cool. Shirt-tail hems fabulously slimming.)

Those were my rules. I would occasionally break them a little, and wear pumpkin-colored hose with my black skirt, for instance. For fun. But for the most part this was it. I worked among designers, otherwise called PIBs (People in Black). So I could get away with a uniform, with wearing black every single day without comment from anyone.

On my run through those wretched stores, I bought everything in my size that fit these requirements. No dressing room, no returns, no membership cards, no-nonsense, no thank you.

After reaching my goal size, I went through a period of trying out newer things, wearing trendy clothes, and shopping in the very tony shops, just because I could. It's been interesting. But where the rather comfortable, rigidly uniformed old me meets a wide-open fashion world, there is much cause for confusion. I miss my boundaries.

My new wardrobe runs far over my old borders to embrace . . . Camel! Tweed! I have patterned pants. They are black-and-white, of course, but definitely patterned. These new items introduce orders of complexity that make me nervous. I find I need a whole wardrobe of belts, shoes, and purses now. A horribly expensive and inefficient way to live, I think.

> There is, for the first time in my adult life, a reasonably direct correlation between my closet and *W* magazine.

I am entering a woman's world. There is, for the first time in my adult life, a reasonably direct correlation between my closet and *W* magazine. That is, I have accessories. I'm trying to go with the flow, but it is a new and strange world full of rules someone else has written for me. I don't understand it. For instance, I now own thongs. But I'm not sure why. If you know, please write and tell me.

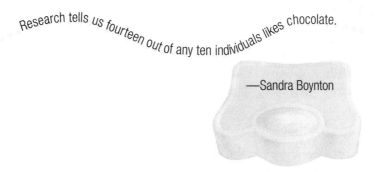

Research tells us fourteen out of any ten individuals likes chocolate.

—Sandra Boynton

The Power of a Dress Size
By Heather Lockwood

The e-mail came out of nowhere. I belonged to an e-mail support group for women competing in a magazine-sponsored fitness challenge. The group basically focused on the topics of fitness, losing weight, and motivation. I didn't participate much. In fact, most of the advice was stuff I had heard before. But the list served as a source of motivation. I felt like if I surrounded myself with health and fitness information 24-7, it was bound to rub off eventually and I'd suddenly make goal or run a marathon or develop an ironclad will, which would make me immune to chocolate chip cookies and hot, buttered toast.

The subject of this e-mail read "Beautiful Women":

Pretty Lady
IT'S BEAUTIFUL WOMEN MONTH & TAG YOU'RE IT!
Did you know that it's Beautiful Women Month?
Well, it is and that means you and me. I'm supposed to send this to
FIVE BEAUTIFUL WOMEN, and you are one of them!!!

Facts on Figures:
- There are 3 billion women who don't look like supermodels and only eight who do.
- Marilyn Monroe wore a size 14.
- If Barbie was a real woman, she'd have to walk on all fours due to her proportions.
- The average woman weighs 144 pounds and wears between a size 12 and 14.

- One out of every four college-aged women has an eating disorder.
- The models in the magazines are airbrushed—not perfect!
- A psychological study in 1995 found that three minutes spent looking at a fashion magazine caused 70 percent of women to feel depressed, guilty, and shameful.
- Models twenty years ago weighed 8 percent less than the average woman. Today they weigh 23 percent less.

***Please send this to at least five phenomenal women today in celebration of Women's History Month.

While it was hokey, and I'd read it in various incarnations over the years, this e-mail, which constituted an exercise in self-validation, was just a reminder that we are better than that. It was a reminder that we, as women, are not completely our outside image. It is bad enough that the media has eroded this belief with years of bombarding us with images of unrealistic women and unrealistic body types. We owe ourselves some reversal therapy. We need to be reminded that we, in our current state, are okay. There is no need to look like the cover of a magazine.

What happened on the list after the initial "Beautiful Women" e-mail went out surprised me. I expected no one to comment, or if anyone did, I thought it would be in joyful agreement. The opposite occurred.

One writer vehemently refuted the idea that Marilyn Monroe was a size 14 at all. In fact, she said, Marilyn was much smaller and exercised. The writer then went on to lambaste Americans for growing in size, clothing makers for responding, and finally, women for using such myths as an excuse for being larger and accepting lower standards. Her tone insinuated that there was something essentially wrong with being a size 14. At the time, I was a size 14.

More discussion ensued among the group's other members: *"Yes, sizes were smaller in the 1940s." "Yes, the American dress size continues to go up and up." "Marilyn Monroe was REALLY a size 10."*

The entire time this went on, my only thought was, what is the fucking point? I kept thinking, "You women are completely missing the point!"

In my mind, the point is, it doesn't matter what size you wear. It doesn't matter what size Marilyn Monroe wore. The point is that Marilyn was curvy and sexy and there is no reason for women to aspire to the size 0 to 2 figures we see plastered on magazines. Finally, there is nothing wrong with a size 14, especially if at size 14 a woman is healthy, fit, and active. I know this is possible. My size 14 was much healthier than the size 0 to 2 women out there who smoke, don't exercise, and binge drink.

Still, none of the e-mail responses addressed this point. Instead, we got an analogy of how a girl who is now a size 4 can finally "flirt" and how she gets compliments from strangers.

If wearing a size 4 means a person can finally flirt with another person, you have to wonder about the power that this number contains. This is a number on a tag on a piece of clothing that isn't even viewable to the outside world. And, yet, it can control a person's attitude.

When I was larger, I invested more emotions in my clothing size. As the label on my pants edged up and up and started straddling the boundaries of regular retail and plus-size chains, I became much more aware of what that number was and who saw it. If I happened to be at the gym, I would fold my clothing over on the bench in an effort to hide the "Women's 16" that seemed to shout from the confines of my cardigan. If a coworker asked my dress size, I'd answer her with a knee-jerk,

> We owe ourselves some reversal therapy. We need to be reminded that we, in our current state, are okay. There is no need to look like the cover of a magazine.

one-size-smaller response. Looking back at this, I am amazed that a simple garment from Liz Claiborne could elicit such lies and deceit from my lips. But that is exactly what it and the rest of my clothing did.

I became overly sensitive as I grew in size, though some of it was ingrained from childhood. I was the girl who was wider than she was tall. Clothing sizes were never easy for me. I recall searching, alongside my mother, through rack after rack of pants trying to locate a size 12 regular or size 12 short instead of the size 12 slim that were in absolute abundance. As a child, most of my pants were too long. They didn't make petites for girls. Worse yet, I'd made the embarrassing transition where my actual clothing size was higher than my age. Changing in gym class, I never wanted my fellow 8-year-olds to see my size 12 knickers that just happened to come below my knees because I was both too short and too wide for those knee-length fashion plates.

I suppose these early experiences with clothing makers were the basis of the love-hate relationship that followed me into adolescence. I hate to admit how much time and energy I spent in high school and college focused on my double-digit sizes when my girlfriends were petite 4s and 6s. These numbers meant a lot. Sizing was something to be proud or ashamed of. And I spent years in search of the perfect brand on the basis of the perfect size. I knew the clothing at Lerner New York was always more forgiving than the Limited. My shopping habits formed solely on the basis of trying to fit into one brand's size 10 jeans.

Somewhere along the line, however, I finally let go. I'm not sure if it was exhaustion or enlightenment or maybe just the fact that I wanted to wear Kenneth Cole even if it meant purchasing a size 16 top. But I gave up on my quest of the lower numbers and I exchanged it for how well the clothes made me feel and reflected in the mirror. There are too many things in this world to get hung up on, and clothing sizes stopped seeming important enough to be one of them.

I do still fall back into old habits. I cannot deny that. As I have lost weight over the past few years, I can't say I haven't delighted in seeing the number on the label of my blouse dip to digits not seen since high school. That is a good feeling. However, I'd like to say the difference now is that *that* isn't the major source of inspiration for me. It is not even part of it. I just want clothing that fits. And I don't care too much if that comes in a medium or small. I just want to approve of my reflection in the mirror, a place where those digits on your clothing never show up.

The writer who launched this heated e-mail debate probably meant no harm. I am sure she was trying to help and was even trying to be motivating in some sort of way. If being skinny has changed her life, I'm happy for her. I'd like to be skinny, too. Now, for me, I equate wanting to be skinny with wanting sparkly purple lip-gloss. It is something I want. It is not something I need.

I need my health. That is why I took charge of my life and started exercising and eating right in the first place. I want to live a long time. I want to be active. And all of that is possible at a size 14, a size 6, a size 12.

The size is arbitrary. Sending a message to a health and fitness support group insinuating anything else is just wrong, especially since most of the people who belong to the group are probably size 14 or larger anyway. Just because a certain person has managed to slim down to a size 4 and is happy she can now flirt doesn't mean she has the right to pass judgment on what sizes are right or wrong for others in the group. That type of attitude is not motivating to anyone; it is insulting. And it is shallow.

One of the last e-mails she sent to the list stated at the end, "Lazy is ugly."

I suppose this is true. But smug is ugly, too. And so is being judgmental. There is nothing out there that states a size 14 is lazy. Nothing.

The Fat Clothes Manifesto
By Shauna Marsh

Some time ago there was an international convention of Fat Clothes Manufacturers (FCM) and they passed a bill that stated:

> *Fat Chicks don't feel bad enough about themselves already, what with the squeezing into small seats and rarely getting laid. So let us strive to make them feel worse by ensuring their quest to be clothed is fraught with maximum misery.*

I have kindly translated their Five-Point Manifesto:

1. Function Not Form

The message from the FCM is clear: You should feel darn lucky we make *any* clothes for you at all, tubby! While the quality and price of plus-size clothing has vastly improved in the United States and Britain, smaller countries like Australia have been slower to capitalize on the Fat Dollar.

I was at my heaviest in the late nineties, when I was starting my first job and looking for a corporate wardrobe. At the lower end of the budget, I could choose shapeless shirts with palm tree prints and team them with flimsy leggings that accentuated the bag-of-potatoes quality of my thighs. If I felt like splashing out, I could buy a frumpy mother-of-the-bride suit, with tapered trousers of course. The FCM largely ignore our cries for quality, affordable pieces in flattering styles.

2. Reflect Not Deflect

Intelligent folks know that matte natural fabrics are the most flattering to a fuller figure—something to skim the body and compliment the curves. But the FCM prefers us to be draped in shiny, violently patterned rubbish. Got a wedding or graduation coming up? Don't expect anything subtle and sexy.

When I was a size 28 I had one Special Occasion Shirt, the only thing I could find in town that looked remotely formal. It was made of some squelchy remnant of a space suit, glistening gold and textured, and splashed with a mutant black rose print. While the cut was decent, the shiny fabric bounced light off every lump and bump, accentuating my loaf-shaped bosom and stopping just short of hanging a "Wide Load" sign on my ass.

"That's very unique," strangers at parties would remark.

"It suits your coloring," my mother said, ever the diplomat.

A formal plus-size purchase also costs at least three times as much as a normal size. So you're stuck with it forever. I glittered my way through two weddings, a christening, and four unsuccessful job interviews.

3. Humiliate and Isolate

Department stores always shove the plus-size collection in the most inaccessible place. In the basement, on the top floor, behind twenty-seven rows of saucepans—whatever makes it the most difficult for the larger lady to make a quick dash in to grab an ill-fitting sack during her lunch hour. What is the reasoning behind this? Perhaps the more remote the location, the less they have to acknowledge that the plus-size section even exists. Or maybe they think, *The walk will do you good, fatty!*

Like an explorer trekking to the North Pole, the epic journey often ends with disappointment. After a fruitless riffle through racks of shapeless sacks, we have to walk all the way back through the store.

Sometimes I swear the racks of skinny clothes are laughing at me as I shuffle past, empty-handed.

4. Dangle a Carrot

The FCM aren't content just to stock plus-size stores with their garish garments. They like to extend their evil influence by collaborating with some so-called Skinny Stores to stock a few token larger sizes that are not bloody large at all. This is done purely to tease the larger lady into thinking that perhaps she could actually buy something young and groovy.

I was the victim of this cruel tactic in Australia. I innocently wandered past a boutique with a sign in the window declaring Sizes 6–20 Available! (US 2–16).

I dared to feel a small coil of hope that I'd find something that didn't make me look like a lumpy schoolmarm. At the time I was 100 pounds down and flushed with newfound confidence. I strolled in and picked up a pair of size 20 jeans, only to try them on and discover I couldn't get them past my knees. I pulled and pulled but they clung to my calves like a tantruming toddler. Ten minutes of hopping and swearing followed as I struggled to disengage in the tiny cubicle. And, of course, the spaghetti-limbed sales staff were on me like a flash when I tried to quietly return them to the shelves: "How were those? Can I get you a different size?"—knowing full well I had reached the upper limit of their range. I slinked out and cried in the car park.

5. Discourage Intimacy

What is the logic behind this one? Are the FCM concerned for their sweatshop employees, and want to spare them the trauma of visualizing fat people getting naked as they sew our gigantic bras?

It's more likely that the FCM simply thinks we do not deserve to have sex, ever. I came to this conclusion while standing beneath the clothesline one sunny morn. As I squinted up, the breeze caught in a row of my giant panties, making them billow like sails. It was a soul-crushing moment. So I have a large rear, but must it be punished and clad in sensible pastel cotton? What's wrong with some sexy fabrics, a scrap of lace, some racy colors? And I don't mean the tarty polyester pap you can order on adult Web sites. I just want to feel feminine and classy. The FCM wants me to have the sex appeal of a cement truck.

But before I can even get down to my knickers, there's the problem of the PJs. Hopefully the market is better in the United States and United Kingdom, but in Australia the chances of sleeping in style are slim. Where are the plus-size pajamas that aren't lilac and don't have a cartoon kitty emblazoned across the chest? Nightgowns are just as horrific—you have a choice of pink or baby blue flannel. Would you like that in plain or floral? Is it any wonder I'm heading to bed with a block of chocolate for company?

I'm all set to start a lobby group to take on the Fat Clothing Manufacturers. We'll write letters, we'll sign petitions, we'll make a bonfire out of giant panties and unflattering capri pants and dance around it *naked* until they start listening to our needs. Who's with me?

> I really don't think I need buns of steel.
> I'd be happy with buns of cinnamon.
> —Ellen DeGeneres

Clothes Talker
By Erin J. Shea

I can't stop thinking about size.

My thought pattern flashes this neon-lit marquee with the words "All Sizes! All the Time!" I'm thinking about my size, your size, her size, and the size of that woman who sits across the room from you at your office. What size is she?

I look at women on TV and in magazines, and I wonder what size they are. Are they a size 2? A size 8? A size 14? Do those women look like me at all? I knew they didn't when I was heavier, but what about now? Could I wear the clothes that they are wearing? And what about my friends? What size are they?

At my heaviest weight, 188 pounds, I would dream about the clothes I could wear once I reached a certain weight. In my head dwelled Malibu Erin and her Dream Closet of Clothes, crammed with dresses that hugged her shape and pants that would sooner be torn into shreds than ride up her crotch. Admittedly, I would play with Malibu Erin and tinker with her weight, trying to ascertain if at 163 pounds she could finally stop wearing pants made of a stretch material. At 151, would she look okay with her shirt tucked in? Glory be—at 135 would it be possible for her to wear whatever she wanted?

Strangely enough, getting Malibu Erin into a pair of jeans when I imagined her at 155 was much easier than when I conjured her up at 135. Imagining a smaller body, and the size and style of clothes that would suit it, was beyond my capacity. I hadn't known such a weight since I first hit puberty.

There are some advantages to having spent the majority of my life being fat, the first of which is that I've always known what looks good on my body. Never did I question whether or not I could pull off a cropped top. Unequivocally, the answer was "no." Even if I wanted a shirt that would expose my midriff, there was no way I'd ever feel comfortable in one, so why waste the money. Sticking to pants that rode just below my waist and blouses that hung mid-thigh masked innumerable sins and I didn't pretend otherwise. Never did I feel ashamed or embarrassed. Not once. Rare was the time when I didn't have something I could wear with poise. I had mastered the art of dressing for my weight.

> Despite owning very little that reflected trends of the day, I truly loved my clothes. Rare was the time when I didn't have something I could wear with poise. I had mastered the art of dressing for my weight.

I owned a fabulous, flouncy black pantsuit that when paired with any number of my silk scarves always earned me rave reviews from strangers and friends alike. It only cost me $40, was a size "XXL," and an important staple of my wardrobe.

Fifty pounds later, I find myself missing that suit. Without a doubt, I knew that when I put it on I looked good. Fifty pounds later, I've lost the ability to tell the difference.

Here is what no one tells you about losing weight: You might wake up one day and wish you were still fat.

For as many rewards that exist to being thin—and there are an obvious multitude such as being in better health, having more energy, even shopping in clothing stores once off-limits to you—there are just as many drawbacks. For me, the scariest of these is that I no longer have a definite idea of what my body actually looks like, let alone what would flatter it most.

This is the first time in my life I've lost weight and kept it off, forcing myself into clothing sizes that in diets of years past I'd wear only once or twice before putting the weight right back on. Unless I want to subject the public at large to my naked glory, I have to buy more than one item in these sizes and in styles that are completely foreign to me. There are few billowy black pantsuits in a size 10. When you're a size 10, they assume you're brave enough for miniskirts and mountains of cleavage. These are not suitable fashion options for a girl who, up until two years ago, could barely see past her belly to her toes when she stood upright in the shower.

> Here is what no one tells you about losing weight: You might wake up one day and wish you were still fat.

March of 2004 found me in the middle of a dressing room at Banana Republic with one of my best friends from college. Wendy offered to accompany me on this trip since I was in dire need of formal clothes and choosing such attire for myself was never my strong suit. After determining that I still wasn't ready for form-hugging dresses, we spotted a pair of cream-colored satin pants. As suggested by our friends at Banana Republic, we checked out a strapless black top made of the same satin material. Hastily I grabbed the pants in a size 12, knowing that formal clothes ran small on me. For the top, I snagged a size 14, as the cut was fitted and I wanted it to hang loosely around my midsection.

Wendy scrunched up her face as I exited the dressing-room stall.

"It looks awful, doesn't it," I asked her.

"Well, yeah," Wendy replied. She paused. "But, Erin, only because it's too damn big on you."

I stared back at her, then proceeded to spin and twist and fidget in front of the three-way mirror. "You think so? I think if I went with a smaller size it wouldn't work the way I want it to," I said.

"Erin, it doesn't work now. You need to try on a smaller size."

Before I knew it, Wendy had summoned the store manager to fetch me a size 10 in the pants *and* the shirt. I returned to the stall and paced the floor, nausea working its way through my entire digestive system. The next noises I heard came from the perky voice of the store manager and the swish from the smaller-sized items being thrown over the stall door.

"Here you go! I brought you some shoes to try with them!"

Slowly I placed one leg, then the other, into the pants and readied myself to maneuver my belly. Sucking in my gut, I slipped the latch of the pants into its hook, pulled up the zipper, and exhaled.

They fit. No extra layers of fat tumbled over the band. The top fit, too. I walked out of the dressing room to stare back at myself in the mirror, the black stiletto heels situated perfectly on my feet, their pointy tips peeking out from the bottom of the pants.

"Now that looks *much* better," Wendy said excitedly. "Didn't I tell you the smaller size would work?"

Only, it didn't work. My reflection in that three-way mirror proved nothing more to me than my ability to wear the smaller sizes. No matter how many times I examined myself in those beautiful pants, ran my hands over their smooth material, walked back and forth from the dressing stall to the tiny room outside of it, the outfit *didn't* work. Searching every place inside myself for another conclusion was fruitless; nowhere could I find the voice that told me *That's really you in that outfit, girl. You are supposed to look like that in those pants, in that top. You can wear it. Go ahead. Buy it.*

Quietly I told Wendy that I didn't want to spend the money on an outfit I would likely wear only once. I placed the pants and top back on their respective hangers, politely thanked the manager for her time, and we left empty-handed.

My body isn't really *my* body anymore. I can make it run faster and longer; if I want, my body will make it through an entire bike ride up and down Chicago's lakefront with nary a whimper. My body can bend and jump, twist and turn in ways it hasn't since I was a teenager. Daily I fuel it with items that nourish me both physically and mentally.

The only thing I can't make my body do is help me identify who I am within it.

When people in my life praise the work I've done with my body, I don't know what to say. I'm no longer certain what it is that they are looking at. Before, I knew what a Fat Girl looked like and I was sure I knew that Fat Girl was who people saw when they looked at me. I knew how to respond. There was great comfort in the face of such certainty.

Each day I wake up praying that I'll hear the voice inside of me giving me permission to accept who I am in a thinner body, in the clothes that it can wear. So far, the dawn is met with silence and I struggle to find something to put on with the same ease and confidence I possessed when wearing those oversized shirts and stretchy pants.

Maybe one day I'll hear that voice. Maybe one day it'll be mine.

> Many of the most virulent stereotypes about women in general have not been discarded but merely transferred, so that negative qualities once attributed to all women are now considered the sole province of fat women.

—W. Charisse Goodman,
The Invisible Woman

Does This Chapter Make Me Look Fat?
By Robyn Anderson

All I wanted when I was a chubby nine-year-old was a T-shirt from the JC Penney catalog, a simple shirt with Mickey Mouse on the front. I was sure that if I got a T-shirt like that, I'd be the coolest kid to hit fifth grade, and people would fall over themselves to be my best friend. Tragically, they didn't make the shirt in my size. As an adult, I assuage that same pain by buying snarky T-shirts whenever I get the chance, and while people don't fall over themselves to be my best friend, I can see the "Who is *that* cool girl?!" in their eyes.

Before I continue, I must confess that I once owned the ugliest shirt ever created, and I include those hideous designs they try to pass off as high fashion. It didn't fit me—it was a size too large—and was a white shirt festooned with multi-colored pistols. Not only did this shirt exist and not only did I actually *buy* it, but there also once existed multiple pictures of me smiling in this shirt as though I had no idea just how horrific it was. Most likely, I didn't. When, years later, I came across the aforementioned pictures, I destroyed them, as any clear-thinking woman would.

I've never been what you might call a fashion plate. When I was little, my mother sewed the majority of my clothes, something I appreciate a great deal now (can you imagine sewing clothes for four ungrateful kids?), but back then I was such a brat that all I wanted was store-bought clothes. When I got older I did get the longed-for store clothes, but shopping was so incredibly boring that if my mother held up an outfit in my size and asked if I'd wear it, I would nod just to get the ordeal over with faster.

When I had my first job and car and could buy my own clothes, I immediately did what I considered the smart thing: I bought all shirts two sizes too large to hide my body. I went through a fluorescent phase (this was the eighties, okay?) wherein I matched oversized fluorescent pink (or green) shirts to fluorescent socks. At that point, I was still small enough that I could shop in the stores for clothes a size or two too big, though later even the Lane Bryant stores didn't carry large enough sizes for me.

At eighteen, I had a great collection of oversized sweaters, which I wore with button-up shirts to further hide my body. In particular, I owned a sweater with thick horizontal stripes across the chest. By all rights, that sweater should have made me look bigger, and while my bust *did* look bigger (though it didn't by any means *need* to), the rest of me looked somehow smaller. Every time I wore that sweater, someone asked if I'd lost weight. I wore that sweater until it was in tatters, and I still miss it a little.

The older I got, the harder it was to find clothes that fit me. Once I was married and pregnant, it was beyond difficult—it was nearly impossible. I don't want to date myself, but it's so much easier now to find clothes that fit you when you're a 26/28 than it was fifteen years ago. Back then, Lane Bryant or Fashion Bug might carry a couple of shirts in that size, but there wasn't a wide selection by any means. I had to resort to buying clothes from the Lane Bryant and Roaman's catalogs. Neither of these catalogs had anything that could be termed fashionable, but all I wanted was to cover my body. And if the clothes were a size or two too big, all the better.

I ordered a denim jumper when I was about six months pregnant, and for the last few months of my pregnancy, I wore that jumper with varying shirts underneath it almost exclusively. By the time I gave birth, my mother was ready to burn the damn thing—in fact, she might have done so; I have no idea what happened to it.

I spent the next ten or so years ordering T-shirts and cotton pants from the catalogs. The shirts sometimes had ugly appliqué designs on the front, or a horrid flowery design all over, but as long as they fit and were comfortable, I was happy (as happy as I could be, anyway). If I by chance stumbled on a shirt I liked in Lane Bryant or Fashion Bug, I'd buy the shirt in every color they had. I once bought a tie-dyed T-shirt that hung down to my thighs, and I felt so anonymous and like no one could tell how fat I was, that I wore it all the time. Just who was I trying to kid? No one looked at me and said "What a thin woman. . . . " Instead, I'm sure they said, "Oh, here comes that fat woman in the tie-dyed shirt. Doesn't she ever wear anything else?"

Don't get me started on bras. I was a hard-to-fit size (a 52DD) and couldn't find anything in any stores. I had to resort to ordering a bra, waiting for it to be shipped to me, trying it on, and returning it for a different size if it didn't fit, over and over until I had what I needed. If I found one I liked and was comfortable (I had a really hard time with bra straps slipping down my arms), I'd order an additional six or seven of them. It was the same with underwear. And once I found bras and underwear that fit, I wore them until they were ragged, then started the whole process over again.

Today, 125 pounds and many sizes down from my highest weight, you'd think I'd be an absolute clotheshorse, but you'd be wrong. I just can't wear clothes that fit me correctly. I can't! I still tend toward T-shirts and cotton pants, and while I'm okay if the cotton pants fit the way they should, I can't feel comfortable wearing a T-shirt that fits properly. I've tried it, believe me, but having the cloth of a shirt actually touch my stomach makes me twitchy and uncomfortable and sooner rather than later I have to go change. I almost never have occasion to dress up, but on the occasion that I do have to attend a concert at my daughter's school, I have a nice, dark tan shirt that works. Sadly, it's the only "nice" shirt I own, though I do have some nice sweaters I can wear in the winter.

At the age of thirty-six, I've spent well over half my life buying clothes solely for the purpose of hiding my body; I'm not sure that that's a habit I'll ever be able—or willing—to change. My favorite piece of clothing is an old yellow nightgown (with an ugly flowered design) that is almost worn to shreds. If I could get away with it, I'd probably wear it all the time. I don't, but it crosses my mind from time to time. I still have the tendency to find a bra that I like, and buy seven more. The same with underwear—I have plain cotton underwear in every color you can imagine. Nothing sexy, no thongs, just plain cotton panties, plain cotton bras. It's nice knowing that if I have to have decent clothes, I can easily find them in my size. I actually own a black dress (though not a *little* black dress) that fits me. I never wear it—I had to buy it for a funeral—but if I needed to, I could. And the clothing industry has stretched enough that even if I were still at my highest weight, I could still find something. It would take work and a lot of shopping, but I could make it happen. Fifteen years ago, I would have been out of luck.

At the age of thirty-six, I've spent well over half my life buying clothes solely for the purpose of hiding my body; I'm not sure that that's a habit I'll ever be able—or willing—to change.

Clothes Make the Girl
By Lori Ford

I've been to Lane Bryant twice in my life. I can't think of another store in history (and trust me, I love to shop) that I know exactly how many times I've visited.

It wasn't until I was in college and living with my first serious boyfriend that I had to face that what were normally my fat clothes—all a size 14—were now too small. However, denial was relatively easy. It's a sign of affection to wear your boyfriend's baggy clothes and since we worked at the same restaurant I could easily wear his "baggy" T-shirts and khaki shorts and not think too much about my size.

One day I was waiting on two cute college boys. When I brought out their drinks one of them said, "You look like that girl on *The Facts of Life*," and snapped his fingers to recall which girl. Horrified, I prayed, please don't say Natalie. "Blair?" I offered.

"You look like that girl on *The Facts of Life*," and snapped his fingers to recall which girl. Horrified, I prayed, please don't say Natalie, please don't say Natalie. . . .

"No, the other one . . . Natalie." And they both looked at me, recognizing her in me. I wanted to cry. I wanted to run and hide from them. They had complete straight faces about it. There was no weight issue or pretty face issue or you should exercise issue. It was just you look like her. That's who you are. They seemed to accept it in me, and I realized that I had accepted my weight as well. It was who I had become.

It was around this time that my boyfriend's shorts were getting tight on me. I had to buy new clothes and there was only one place I knew of where I'd be able to find something that fit.

Lane Bryant.

I enlisted the help of my boyfriend's overweight sister. I needed a reassuring brave face to help find simple khaki shorts for work. Someone had to get me in and out of there quickly and without being noticed by anyone. It was the early 1990s, so I suppose the bright colors, large patterns, and sticky rayon/polyester blends shouldn't have affected me so much, but immediately I was lightheaded and craved a very large brownie. My boyfriend's sister took me straight over to the shorts and I grabbed a few smaller-sized pairs, immediately telling myself, *Well, you're a small size here, and when was the last time you were perusing the smaller-sized stuff, the front of the rack, not digging in desperation for the back of the pile, disrupting the Gap's carefully folded table displays to get to the XLs?"*

In the dressing room I found out I was a size 18 and I started crying. It was like I got a really bad haircut. I was looking at myself in bad lighting, and I was ugly. I was huge. I was a plus size. As I left with my size 18 khaki shorts, I swore I'd never cross a Lane Bryant store threshold again.

When my boyfriend and I split up shortly thereafter I returned home and lost 70 pounds. I maintained, give or take 20 pounds, for quite a while. Then one day I seemed to lose all hope in myself and my size 14s again became tight. I needed an outfit for a Christmas party. The Gap had nothing dressy enough for me to wear. Lane Bryant had recently had a terrific image overhaul. The images of plus-sized models on the posters leaping out the front doors of the shop were beautiful and sexy and the clothes looked attractive on their disturbingly flat size-16 tummies. Certainly there'd be something for me in a size 14 or maybe a size 16 that I could find for the party. Almost ten years after my previous vow, I crossed into Lane Bryant's store again, trying to feel normal, trying to feel like a girl, trying not to break down in tears.

I was approached by a beautiful, voluptuous girl wearing a snazzy wide-scarf headband. I thought to myself, *I could be stylish and adorable like her.* I wanted something simple. A simple, straight black skirt, knee-length, made with natural fibers and a button-down white shirt preferably with slimming princess seams. I passed a rack of large stringy corsets as the salesperson hunted down a simple black skirt. The best she could find was a rayon blend black skirt with sequins down the side. Okay. She also found a white shirt with the specifications that I wanted but again it was a bit on the sticky, unbreathable fiber side. I approached the Crying Room, I mean, *the dressing room,* to try on my items.

The skirt looked like a black box hanging at my chubby knees, making my hips and legs seem wider; the sequins drew attention to me, something I was trying to avoid. The shirt didn't look tailored and refined but ill-fitted and blobbish. It washed out my now-drained, pale, horrified face. It was also unmercifully hot. I felt the tears bubbling up. I needed an outfit for the party. What other option did I have? I bought the outfit and vowed never to return to the store again. I was uncomfortable and of ill mood at the party. I longed to be home in PJs eating a pint of ice cream and watching movies.

Again I lost the weight. Got down again to size 6/8. Again I started gaining weight. Some clothes can be worn longer than their intended size, after all. Stretchy pants with stretchy waistbands can be worn as long as you can pretend your panty line isn't showing and the increasing tightness is the style. I have tracksuits that I've worn since gaining 30 pounds. Clothing meant to sling around my hips, especially skirts, have managed to creep up and are now better suited to my waist. I own a skirt with this funny poof about it; the poof is intended to house my butt, but now the skirt rides up so high that the poof is situated on the small of my back. A longer T-shirt will hide it for the most part.

I continue to try to purchase clothing as I make my way up the double-digit sizes, trying not to cross Lane Bryant's threshold again. I've reached the stage where it's just a mess. Size 12s and 14s are cut for tall, thin women, not overweight girls of average height. I'm too tall for petite clothes and they're often cut for thin women as well. Low-rise pants are the style and it's difficult to wear with a stomach seeping over the waistband. It's uncomfortable and not attractive. I can't imagine much of the world's population can wear this cut. Shirts and T-shirts are cut shorter and narrower. I have the most difficulty finding T-shirts and tank tops that don't cling at my stomach and upper arms. I don't want a boy-cut T-shirt. I want a feminine cut that doesn't cling. It's impossible to find. The last time I tried on pants, they clung severely to my thighs and flared impossibly across the floor. It wasn't a matter of being too small; my thighs were simply too large. I can't tell where skirts are supposed to hit me. I've tried on various sizes only to have none of them work for my shape, subsequently falling on me in various places along my torso and hips. The results are skirts too tight, skirts that showcase my stomach bulge, and shirts so expansive that my legs are optional accessories, as you couldn't see them under all of that material.

All the while, these are temporary clothes I'm shopping for. This diet thing will be kicking back in at any moment.

Never order food in excess of your body weight.
—Erma Bombeck

Tarpaulin Is the New Black
By Monique van den Berg

For a while now, I've been experiencing the glories of shopping at "skinny people" stores. I no longer have to head straight for the "Women's" section at the department store or sneak into the Avenue to find a pair of jeans. The days when I had to paw through racks full of hideously ugly clothes in search of one or two acceptable items are over.

Fatty-clothes shopping is a nightmare. First, there's the trauma of having to squeeze your spacious ass through narrow aisles and between crowded racks of clothing. *Then* you go into the dressing room and find that you've picked up something a size too small, and the words *camel* and *toe* suddenly come to mind. *Then* you suffer the indignity of handing everything back to the person handing out clothing tags, who asks, "Did everything work out for you?" and you just know that, looking at you, she's thinking, *Of course nothing fit that giant cow. I wonder if she knows that the Dress Barn is next door?*

The indignity goes on. The fluorescent lights. The "Can I get this in a size"—*whisper*—"eighteen?" The changing rooms that are too small. The sad conviction that the store mannequins—plastic people with no heads—are sexier than you are.

Or the worst: trying on clothes with a skinny friend. Recently I made the mistake of going shopping with a friend of mine from work, who is one of the most beautiful people I have ever met in real life. When a woman who is *seven months pregnant* looks better in everything than you do, it's very demoralizing.

I'm sure you have a friend like this. You try on a top that you think is sort of cute. And then she puts it on and she looks like a supermodel. She buys twenty-seven tops and skirts and pants because *everything looks fabulous on her*, and you end up buying a pair of socks, which is the only thing that you can possibly buy and feel good about.

Do not shop with friends like this.

Outside of the fitting room, you can each be beautiful in your own, unique, special snowflake type of way. Inside the fitting room, you need permission to have fat rolls. And I don't mean beautiful sexy curves, either. You need permission to splooge.

I remember life before I knew Lane Bryant existed. I remember shopping for a prom dress when I was in high school and a size 16. My mother and my grandmother dragged me to twenty stores, none of which carried dresses in my size. Instead, I had to suffer the pain of asking for the "biggest size you have" and then not fitting into it. Why didn't you just take me to the Fatty Store, Mom?

Maybe she (a woman who doesn't shop for clothing and has in fact been wearing the same three outfits since 1972) didn't know that these stores existed. Maybe she was trying to "motivate" me to diet away my baby fat. Maybe she had a secret sadistic streak. Who knows? But I remember that day vividly. I remember buying the one and only dress I fit into, a white wedding dress confection of tulle and lace that I didn't even like. But it was the white monstrosity or no prom. And so I sucked in my stomach, squeezed myself into that dress like frosting into a Twinkie, and went to the prom. As much as shopping for clothes sucks when you're overweight, it's comforting to know that Lane Bryant—these days a source of plus-sized clothing that is

> Fatty-clothes shopping is a nightmare. . . . The sad conviction that the store mannequins—plastic people with no heads— are sexier than you are.

often stylish and cute—exists. Because most Fatty Clothes are a horror. A nightmarish horror from which there is no awakening.

"We know you've given up," says the fashion industry. "Here's a tarp we've covered with flowers and cut a neck hole in. Ponchos are very stylish this season! Or not. What do *you* care?"

And the catalogs! Most of them feature skinny models; they can't even throw the plus-sized models a bone. And they dress these tiny women in clothes that obviously no one in their right mind would wear, unless they were my mother, Bea Arthur, or Mrs. Roper from *Three's Company*. It's just a parade of hideous clothing, and it's all a girl can do to find a simple black tank top without an appliqué sequined starfish on it, or beaded American-flag breast pockets, or some such shit.

> "We know you've given up," says the fashion industry. "Here's a tarp we've covered with flowers and cut a neck hole in. Ponchos are very stylish this season!"

Do you know what I saw the other day? A sweatshirt with a kitten on it. That's not so bad, right? Well, the kitten had green sequins for eyes. Still not so bad? It was wearing a leopard-spotted bandana. Which was made from a piece of fur hot-glued to the front of the shirt. And it was probably from the home-shopping network. *And why is it that only fat people wear clothing like this?*

I can proudly say that I haven't worn a kitten sweatshirt since the age of six. These days, I can expand my horizons.

It's all still very new, though. I go into designer shops and head straight for the accessories section. I want the people in there to know that I know my place—browsing purses and sunglasses, not looking fruitlessly through racks of clothes that come in small, medium, and extra-small. Occasionally I get brave and try something on. I almost fit into a medium the other day at Anthropologie. At H&M, I tried on a generous-looking size 12 shirt and it fit me. And I'm not afraid to shop at Banana Republic anymore, since the extra-large there is often too big on me. (The moment when I found that out was a revelation. It didn't even occur to me that I might look weird in a shirt because it was too big. Me, in a large? I could hardly believe it.)

I can't shop everywhere, but I'm getting closer.

I can always order clothes online in the latest styles; frequently the Web sites carry more sizes than the stores do. (It turns out that if I'd tried, I could possibly have been doing this all along. Not done this sort of self-imposed segregation act and restricted myself to Lane Bryant until I was too skinny for their smallest jeans.)

Anyway, now I shop where all the skinny girls shop. And it's ridiculous. Clothing and fabrics and sizing—the whole messy industry—it's not an exact science. I have to keep reminding myself of that. I try not to be too hard on myself. I enjoy the process of trying on crazy things once in a while and surprising myself when I realize that, hey, off-the-shoulder really *does* look good on me. I really *can* pull off the 1980s Pat Benatar look! (Maybe I'm not surprising myself there so much as deluding myself. Whatever.)

But it sucks that the "skinny" stores don't carry extended sizes. It sucks that I feel like a criminal checking to see if a particularly cute item comes in an extra-extra-large, or if the fabric stretches. And when I take something in and try it on, only to find that the largest size doesn't fit, it sucks that I still feel like a fifteen-year-old who might not get to go to the prom.

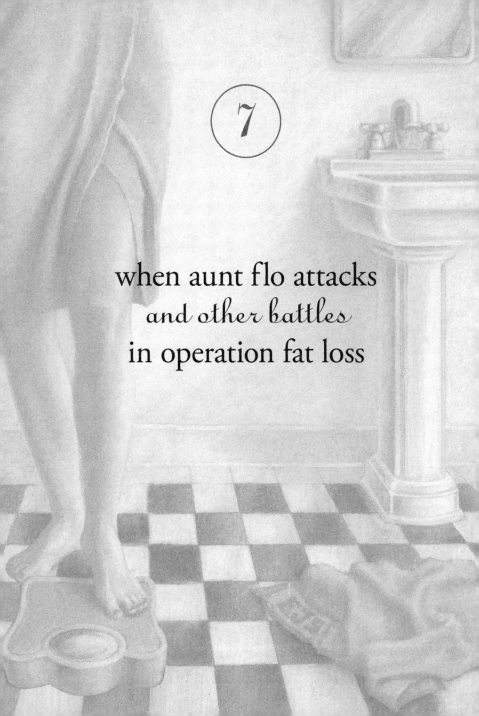

7

when aunt flo attacks
and other battles
in operation fat loss

Flee, Freshman Fifteen!

College is the hardest place to lose weight. It might seem like a comfortable, cushy time of life, but in reality? Grades, a social life, and sleep are like a juggling act. Adding a weight-loss plan can make it feel like you'll drop all the balls.

Whether you're at a large state school or a tiny private institute, weight loss is still tricky. For instance: the gym.

There are two types of people there. I call them the whippets and the jocks. Jocks run on the treadmills and blast heavy metal in the weight room. Whippets, on the other hand, are the tiny girls who spend an hour on the treadmill every day, and don't drink water because it will make them bloat. They frighten me. Food, and all the assorted issues that come with it, tends to be the bane of any college-aged Fat Girl existence. All food comes from the dining hall. One hall claims to cater to a number of lifestyles, with vegetarian and vegan food, a deli, a salad bar, and many other fine choices.

By Naomi Guiterrez

We've all heard how bad college food is. Everything is cooked in buckets of grease. Or filled with heavy cream. I'd eat more from the salad bar, but they consistently serve vegetables that are tasteless, rotting, or otherwise unfit for human consumption. I eat a lot of chicken—at least it's grilled. Atkins would really not work on a college campus.

Plus, it's just hard to eat healthily. If you're at dinner with six people and everybody goes and gets soft-serve from the machine that's so cleverly placed by the salad bar, and you're just sitting there all by your lonesome. And there are never cups by the water and juice machines, but there are always cups by the soda. And on and on.

Between junk food at every turn, a lack of healthy alternatives, and unfriendly facilities, it's enough to make a girl lose hope. The worst part, though, is that nobody expects you to be on a path toward healthiness. It's college. You're supposed to stay out and party and sleep late and eat gross food and drink and gain the "freshman 15" and not think about diets or exercise or any of it. Everybody who comes into my room and sees my scale is honestly surprised to see that I have one. I'm in college! I shouldn't be getting up at six in the morning to go to the gym! But I am. And honestly, I think I'll be happier, and healthier, in the end.

The Sugar Borg
By Julie Ridl

I'm sitting here, post-Christmas chaos, in my new PJs and my new slippers, between a pile of wrapping flotsam and a teetering tower of tins full of shortbread, sugar cookies, fudge, and nut brittles.

You would never know, visiting us this morning after Christmas, that ours is a family constantly working to cut back on added sugars in our diet.

I spoke with a reporter the other day. She asked me how we manage food in our household and how I personally manage food to maintain my 100-pound weight loss and fight off diabetes. I told her when sweet foods come into the house, I ask my husband to help me by removing them or hiding them. Sometimes I can pitch the food myself, but many times I need my husband's diabolical mind and his access to ravenous students to move the supply to areas of demand.

The reporter, being a writer and a muckraker, and naturally thin, leaped on that passive expression. "How," she asked, "do sweet foods 'come into the house'?"

And I was both surprised that she had to ask (doesn't sugar just show up in everyone's lives all the time?) and a little troubled at my inability to put my finger on the actual source of the stuff. Sweet things seep in under the door. My family sneezes cookies. Friends shed sugar all over the floor. It shows up, okay? It does. It just does.

I didn't bake this year. Didn't use sugar or flour at all to make any holiday treats. I didn't actively decide to do this. I held out to the possibility that I would get around to it, but I ran out of time, and chose sleep over the late-night baking binges of years past.

I thought it would be hard to skip baking and not have anything to feed well-wishers and droppers-in. And, well, frankly, baking is one of the few things I do really well. Family recipes, like my killer ginger marmalade rugelach now exist in memory only. Truffles went undipped. I made none of it.

And yet, here I am, sitting in the shadow of this leaning tower of treats. I'd say, pound for pound, there's as much sugar in my house this year as in any year past. Creamy fudges, salty-sweet buckeyes, almond cookies, sugar cookies, twists, sprinkles, mints, and more. Whether people feel sorry for my husband, or this is residual payback for years past, I'm not sure, but in my most passive year ever, the sweet stuff has appeared. How? Who is responsible? Should I have put a sign on the door? Issued warnings in my Christmas cards? Well, when I get around to sending Christmas cards, I mean?

> Maybe sugar is its own force, a higher form of hive intelligence blanketing our planet like a fungus. Perhaps it carries a collective intelligence, and an intention that is not as sweet as its presentation.

Am I even asking the right question? Hey, wait a minute. Why do we assume sugar is inanimate at all? We have always assumed it. But perhaps that's our mistake. We naive humans. Silly ancient species stuck on simple cause and effect.

Maybe sugar is its own force, a higher form of hive intelligence blanketing our planet like a fungus. Perhaps it carries a collective intelligence, and an intention that is not as sweet as its presentation. This would explain so much. It would explain the way it multiplies and changes form to disguise itself (high fructose corn syrup, fruit syrups, brown rice syrup, cane syrup, and all those things ending in -*ose* and -*ol*). It would explain how it moves world economies, jumps oceans, mulches humans, puffing them up before breaking them down. We are one fermenting, bubbling planet, probably soon to become a bon-bon stuffed in some geometrically larger galactic being's holiday tin.

And our house is a target. The more we try to fight this onslaught, the more concentrated the Borganistic bubbling fungus becomes. It started around Halloween, dribbling from the ceiling in dollops and chunks, with the flow picking up considerably by Thanksgiving, and cresting in a near-avalanche yesterday. *EeeeeEEEeee!!!*

> We are one fermenting, bubbling planet, probably soon to become a bonbon stuffed in some geometrically larger galactic being's holiday tin.

And there it is, this tower of stuff, staring at me through its beady buckeyes, in its mute intention to eat me alive, sure of its superior intellect, confident that its prevalence makes fighting against it futile. Lower your shields and surrender your ship. You will be assimilated.

Ah, but I have something the sugar Borg doesn't have. I have my will. Or I did have. It's around here somewhere. It's under the wrapping paper, or perhaps stuffed in a closet somewhere. But it's here.

I'm going to shake it off. I'm going to press out the wrinkles in my willpower and put it on again, good as new. And I'm going to save my family and myself from this sugar infestation.

Ready to fight the good fight?

Man is born to eat.

—Craig Claiborne

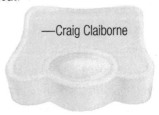

Even Superstars Need Help
By Heather Lockwood

I have to admit something. I've always considered myself a weight-loss superstar. As egotistical as that sounds, it is the truth. I was a Fat Girl. I had my Fat Girl issues. But I conquered them. I started exercising. I became an athlete and I lost 30 pounds.

When I started my journey, I was nearing 180 pounds. And within a couple of years (it didn't come off that fast), I was down in the 150s. The changes I made were lifestyle changes. I became an avid exerciser. I changed my eating habits to include more fruits and vegetables, more organics, and more whole-grain based foods. But other than that, I did what I wanted. I didn't join Weight Watchers. I didn't do Jenny Craig. I didn't even see a nutritionist. At best, I read a lot. I came upon my efforts from more of a health approach than a weight-loss one and, even as the weight came off, I maintained that that wasn't my focus. My focus wasn't to get skinny; it was to get healthy. And I was a superstar.

Of course, I was lying a bit, too. Even though health was my main focus, deep down I wanted to be skinny. But because the weight was coming off so easily, I didn't worry about the being skinny thing because I figured it would eventually just happen. Just like the weight loss eventually happened. All good things in time, right? Right.

Then at some point when I hit my lowest weight of around 147, my body settled. And there I was for a long, long time.

Week after week, I weighed myself. I went through the routine: empty bladder, remove shoes, step on scale. And week after week, I made no progress.

So there I was in the upper 140s. And there I started on a three-year plateau. Yes, that's right: a three-year plateau. It is then that I started asking myself, who's the superstar now?

But I knew the drill. I forged ahead. And I continued about my life with my healthy, superstar habits, hoping this temporary stall was just that, temporary. But as the weeks turned into months and the months turned into years, it began to dawn on me that unless something became drastically different, that scale was not going to move.

I can't even begin to explain how frustrating this was because, according to the books, I was doing everything right. I had all the answers. What could I possibly be doing wrong? I exercised six to eight hours a week. I made menus of healthy meals that I religiously posted on my refrigerator. I read each issue of all my fitness magazines from cover to cover, nodding all along the way. I knew this stuff. Snack on carrots at work: check. Feel hungry, take a walk: check. Get awesome abs by using the ball workout twice a week: check. Drink your water: check. Take your vitamin: check. Eight hours of sleep: CHECK.

> My focus wasn't to get skinny; it was to get healthy. And I was a superstar.

Or did I? From time to time, that question would creep into my head, mostly at times like when I hopped up from my office chair to unwrap a few pieces of chocolate from the office candy stash. But the question hurt too much to answer. I deserved this chocolate because I was a superstar. Everything else I did was perfect. Besides, we can't deprive the superstar, can we? And that is when my cover started to form. If the weight wouldn't budge, my attitude could.

The new attitude was this: I was happy at my weight. Therefore, I was maintaining. I didn't need to lose any more.

So, this is what I preached on the outside. This was my cover. And it was believable. I preached it online. I preached it offline. And, even now,

I still think it is a healthy approach. I had conquered the hard part, the close-to-obesity part. And if most of the American population would do just that, we'd be so much better off.

No, the only problem with this rationale was that it wasn't particularly honest. As much as I told everyone I was happy where I was, I secretly wished for more. I was lying. And as I read diet blog after diet blog, I found myself contemptuous of those who had lost more weight than I had. As my weight stayed firmly planted (and even crept up a few pounds to 150), I followed women online who had started at weights higher than my starting weight, and I watched them dip down to below my current weight. It seemed that everywhere I looked, everyone was losing, everyone except for me. And as much as the whole diet-blogging community is great and can make a dieter—or should I say "Health Enthusiast"—feel less alone, I never felt more acutely different than I did during my plateau.

What was the most disturbing was that I couldn't (or wouldn't) understand it. It didn't make sense to me because I wasn't eating at McDonald's. I wasn't committing all those normal dieting faux pas. In fact, I was exercising like a fiend. My pantry was stocked with low-fat, high-fiber nuggets of goodness. I had the tools. I was using the tools.

And yet, the weight stayed the same.

The more frustrated I became, the more I exercised. I even started logging my food into FitDay.com, a free online source for calorie counting. I set a target range for myself that I halfheartedly hit. All the while, I maintained that I was maintaining. I saved face by convincing others that 150 was my ideal weight because that is where my body, obviously, wanted to be.

Still, I'd troll the Internet and read over and over stories about lovely ladies reaching a size 10 and finally dipping into the 130s. I managed to filter out all of those accounts from those who where struggling much like myself. It was the successes that would stick with me and make me green with envy. As much as I publicly stated I was happy where I was, I wasn't. I wanted to lose more.

In hindsight, it is no surprise that my weight stayed constant. There were key factors that I refused to examine during these three years, factors like the office chocolate and an extra glass of wine to two with dinner. And I simply didn't want to face the fact that my body needed change. That, for me, to lose more weight, I needed to do more. I'd hit the peak capacity that I was going to hit with my calories-in to calories-out ratio. As successful as this superstar was at losing 30 pounds by eating pretty much whatever she wanted, it wouldn't continue. It simply couldn't continue.

I accepted the fact that perhaps I didn't know everything. And within a week I started to lose weight.

So, the superstar wasn't such a superstar after all.

Sometimes hubris is the biggest obstacle of all.

Recently, I was able to face this demon. I just got tired of lying and asserting to the world that I was happy at my current weight when, the truth was, I wasn't. I had to face the fact that I didn't hold all the answers. If I did, I wouldn't be so unhappy.

But hardest of all, I had to face the fact that I had changed. I was now different from the Fat Girl I once was. I also was different from all the diet bloggers that I read. So, I couldn't use their answers. The same thing that can cause Person A to lose weight may not do jack for me. So, as motivating as diet journals can be, I needed to stop comparing myself so directly. I couldn't use anyone else's formula but my own. And, more importantly, I needed to figure out what that formula was. Finally, I needed to get down off my superstar throne and start looking for answers.

In the end, I did something that the superstar never would have done. I asked for help. I let go of my know-it-all attitude and I started a diet program, something I once said I would never do. I accepted the fact that perhaps I didn't know everything. And within a week, I started to lose weight.

Since joining the program, I have had the opportunity to step back and recognize my mistakes. I let my ego get in the way and I never asked for help. I simply did not want to admit that I was doing something wrong. But now that I have, it is so much easier to rely on someone else's know-how. Handing over that trust and work allows me to better assess what works and what does not. It is amazing how releasing control can give you so much more.

I know there will be future obstacles that I will still have to tackle in this journey. I will make mistakes. I will need to seek help to correct them. But as long as I know I am capable of making these mistakes, I also know I will be capable of conquering them. Sometimes being aware of our faults can be the greatest asset of all.

"Probably nothing in the world arouses more false hopes than the first four hours of a diet."

—Dan Bennett

Binge 101
By Shauna Marsh

I didn't always know how to binge. It was a skill that I picked up, much in the same way you learn to ride a unicycle or play the sitar. Only binging is an infinitely easier task.

I got my first Binge Lesson when I started college. My teacher was a girl I knew from high school. She needed a place to live for a few weeks and I had a spare room. So, in she came with the most enormous pile of groceries I'd ever seen. At that point I was around 220 pounds, quite overweight indeed; but I'd been having healthy stir-fries for dinner and had already lost a few pounds.

"We must celebrate tonight!" my new roomie declared. "Let's watch *Felicity* and have a pig-out!"

"Right on," I said. So off we went to the supermarket.

My definition of a pig-out at that time was buying a small packet of chips or maybe a Mars Bar. This is why I'd stayed "manageably fat." As we wandered up and down the aisles, I wondered if I'd choose chips or chocolate tonight. Meanwhile, the roomie was deciding between two different packets of chocolate cookies.

Oh right, I thought, *cookies it is.* I headed for the checkout.

But then she plucked a giant bag of corn chips off a shelf, and then purposefully strode to the dairy section where she selected a tub of French onion dip. A family-size block of Cadbury's Dairy Milk Chocolate was the finishing touch.

I was so stunned, I couldn't speak. I couldn't believe she was buying all these things all at once. It had never occurred to me that this could be done.

We got home and parked ourselves in front of the telly. I felt strangely excited as we ripped open the chips and cookies. We shoved two spoons into the ice cream like triumphant astronauts planting flags on the moon. I loved the rustle of foil and paper as I snapped the chocolate bar in half.

Finally, there was no one here to tell me to *slow down with that dip* or to have *one cookie only* or to ration out a single square of chocolate. I was delirious. I'd never eaten ice cream from the tub before. I relished the explosion and texture of cramming a handful of chips into my mouth at once. I followed it up with the creamy grittiness of the ice cream, the salty sweet of a Tim Tam cookie. Forget taking drugs or graffiti-ing my name across the school playground: *this* was rebellion, baby! We ate and ate until the flavors blurred and we couldn't move.

I felt high.

Soon the roomie got a place on campus and she moved out and moved on. But I didn't. That night was a turning point. After that I was on my rapid path to obesity.

Initially it started with the occasional binge like I'd had with the roomie, but then my days became one continual feast. When I arrived at university, I was shy and full of loathing for my already lardy body, so I created a comforting world for myself where it was just me and the food. I drew a strange kind of happiness out of it. Eating became my number-one leisure activity. I'd spend my day secretly planning my feasts, pondering what I would eat next and how I'd get it. As soon as my new roommate left for the weekend to see her folks, I'd drive the three blocks to the supermarket and stock up. Something savory—usually chips and dip or a loaf of white bread and a jar of the Kraft cream cheese spread I'd loved as a child but that Mum only allowed us to have as a treat. *Well, screw you, Mum,* I'd think. *I'm going to toast that loaf and plow my way through the whole jar.*

I always counterbalanced the savory course with something sweet. I had a penchant for Cadbury's Black Forest (family size, of course), Nestlé bar and bagfuls of chocolate-coated honeycomb. I'd buy a jar of Nutella and finish it in one sitting. Then there was the ice cream. I really went to town with that Cookie Cream Commotion; many times I'd eat the entire pint at once then wonder why I felt so ill afterward.

Sometimes I'd do the fast-food binge. My town had a McDonald's, KFC, and Red Rooster on the same block. I'd have a craving for a Red Rooster Hawaiian pack—BBQ chicken, fries, pineapple, and a banana fritter. I'd go to the drive-through for that, ignoring the way my belly was closing in on the steering wheel. Next, I'd think, *I'd love some coleslaw with that*, so I'd go to KFC, as the coleslaw was better there. I'd throw a newspaper over the Red Rooster so the pimply kid on drive-through wouldn't think I was a pig. Then I'd often make a last stop at McDonald's for a chocolate shake or a sundae. Or both. You gotta have dessert.

I would go home and eat it all, quickly and urgently, barely tasting a thing. It was more about the texture of the food, the stringiness of the chicken, the warmth I'd feel as this horrible greasy shit filled up my insides. It was the crunch of the chips, the salt on my fingers, the way the ice cream slid down my throat and made everything feel all cool and calm inside my rib cage. The whole shopping and eating process made me feel purposeful; it was an event. It felt intimate and soothing.

This went on for five years. I gained over 120 pounds.

I've lost all that weight now, plus more, and the Binge behavior is largely under control. I've taught myself to occupy my life with people and hobbies so I don't turn to food to pass the time.

Sometimes when things aren't going well, I'll find myself in the supermarket, absentmindedly picking up something savory, something sweet, and something cold to wash it all down. It scares me how the old habits lurk just beneath the surface.

A Simple Plan
By Erin J. Shea

So I get this little envelope in the mail two weeks ago and in it is a booklet promising a "weight-loss and exercise plan [I] can live with."

I am a chump for plans of any sort, so I excitedly opened this booklet, ready to unlock the secrets of weight loss and exercise that I so obviously have been kept in the dark about. You must understand that despite years of dieting, I remain convinced that someone is holding out on me, just waiting for the right time to reveal him or herself to me and hand over the answer to my problems.

According to the booklet, the first thing I am instructed to do is to "cut calories." What a *great* idea! Why didn't I think of that before?

It isn't the suggestion of cutting calories that I take issue with, but rather the method by which I'm to accomplish this: "Lose one pound a month by simply replacing that regular candy bar with an orange and a banana, or bag the chips and instead have ½ cup of steamed broccoli." Really. Are they kidding? I don't *regularly* eat candy bars or chips, and just reading this sentence makes me want to knock over the vending machine in my office cafeteria to sniff a bag of Fritos.

Every day at 10:30 A.M. and 3:30 P.M., like clockwork, I need to eat. Perhaps it's all of those plans and guides I've read that have conditioned me like the little Pavlov dog that I am, but it's true. Come 10:30 A.M. on Day One of the plan, I partake in a feast of the suggested orange and a banana.

They suck. They really and truly suck. First of all, I have forgotten to pack a knife, which means I had to rip apart my orange with my finger-nails, ruining my manicure and causing the majority of the juice to go spraying onto my monitor, onto my paperwork, and all over my hands. I am left to eat limp wedges of pulp, most of which never even make it past the gaps in my teeth to my stomach, and I spend an inordinate amount of time using whatever I can find trying to pry out the remains because I didn't count on needing a toothpick. As for the banana, well, it was okay. But it's hard to get worked up about a fruit that can so obviously be improved upon by mashing it into a pile of flour, sugar, eggs, chocolate chips and setting the oven to 350 degrees to bake.

By 3:30 P.M., when it's time to eat my ½ cup of broccoli, it's flaccid and a greenish color more suitable to sewer sludge. Plus, the smell is so rank the only thing can I think to do is flush it squarely down the toilet.

Bye-bye, broccoli. Alas, I knew ye well.

The next bit of advice is to "graze; don't gorge." This step wants me to eat four mini-meals each day. I eat a sound breakfast of steel-cut oatmeal and coffee, packing at least two other mini-meals into my lunch sack. One is the meal I plan to have at 10:30 A.M., and since we know that the orange and banana trick didn't bring down the house, I bring a whole-wheat mini-pita and a carefully measured portion of hummus, drizzled with some olive oil. My cupboards are woefully bare, so I decide that I'll run to Subway at lunch for a veggie sub. At 3:30 P.M. I will have an apple and, as suggested, some peanut butter.

The pita and hummus go over much better than the fruit and don't require utensils of any sort. But by 11:30 A.M., I'm still hungry and lunch is another two hours away. I make a mad dash for the refrigerator and my apple and peanut butter.

My lunch break rolls around and I pick up my sub, only to realize I have no 3:30 P.M. snack. I go back and buy a bag of baked potato chips and commence with the sub consumption. As of 1:39 P.M., I am done with the sub and decide to just go ahead and eat the chips.

I crawl through the rest of the day and by 3:23 P.M., I can't help but notice how my stomach seems to be devouring its own lining. When I get home, I order a pizza with a side of Buffalo wings.

Now I'm sitting at home, sucking up the remaining hot sauce from my fingernails when I read the next step on the plan: "snack every four hours." Didn't they just tell me to eat four mini-meals? Isn't there a substantial difference between "meal" and "snack?" Was I supposed to eat these meals on top of the snacks?

Who has time for this much eating? If I break it down logically to fit within all of the hours of my day, I'm infringing on mini-meal time with snack-time. If I don't work in snack time, precisely every four hours, surely I will screw this up. How am I ever going to learn to eat like a normal person if my weight-loss plan calls for me to turn into the White Rabbit from *Alice in Wonderland*?

The meal plan's next tip has to be the work of someone with all of the personality of a wet dishrag: "add lemon zests to fruit and frozen yogurt." Nice. Because we all know what a fitting substitute *lemon zest* is for Cool Whip and chocolate syrup. Appetizing, too!

Following the lemon zest revelation is this one: "Eat Slowly." It takes up to twenty minutes for signals from the stomach to reach the brain. Put the fork down in between bites, focus more on conversation, take small bites, and wait fifteen minutes before taking seconds." This seems like an obsessive-compulsive disorder waiting to happen. Also, the author of these tips has never had a meal with my friends or family. You wait that long, provided everyone else is eating at his or her normal pace, and *then* decide you want another helping, you're out of luck. The food is gone. People are clearing off the table while you're still sitting there focusing on conversation, leaving all to wonder why you not only keep putting your fork down but also why you are carrying on an intense tête-à-tête with yourself.

The plan goes on to tell me more, about how I should incorporate exercise into my daily routine and how I should be more conscious of my food choices. I agree with *these* tips; they're tangible and less aggressive. However, I've decided to toss the booklet and the rest of the magazines with similar plans where they belong: in the trash.

There exists a cacophony of opinions as to how to go about losing weight, more specifically the day-in, day-out minutiae of how weight loss happens. For some, I'm sure these tips work. I'm just not convinced that substitution and anal-retentive attention to food portions is helping me attack the cravings, and I don't foresee myself being able to incorporate any of these tips into my life.

After a couple of days of following this latest plan, I don't feel any healthier. I only feel like a failure and I am tired of failing.

> When you want food—junky, fatty, salty, substantive food—there is no herbal tea that you can dunk into boiling hot water that will be a surrogate for an order of cheese fries.

Mostly I'm tired of the feeling that I have to handle food as though it's a ticking time bomb ready to explode and end up as 20 extra pounds on my ass.

I've read that when you're hungry, you should make a cup of tea. I tried tea. Let me tell you something: Hot tea is *not* a substitute for food. Who are the people who come up with these things? Even more curious to me are the people who follow this advice. Are they Stepford dieters? When you want food—junky, fatty, salty, substantive food—there is no herbal tea that you can dunk into boiling hot water that will be a surrogate for an order of cheese fries. There just isn't. Anyone who looks at you with a straight face and a pair of size 4 jeans and says otherwise is an asshole.

I'm not so insensitive that I don't realize that for some people certain foods are trigger points and that just eating a single bite of those foods can send them into a spiral of diet destruction, so they search high and low for alternatives to these foods.

But I have to wonder: *Aren't most of us really just substituting one neurosis for another?* If I end up plowing through a couple of tasteless, spongy, fat-free cookies when a single chocolate chip cookie might have done the job, how I am better off? How did we all lose such faith in ourselves that we've come to accept that we're powerless in the face of a chocolate craving, so we eat this *faux food* and pretend to be thankful for it? What did we do with our self-worth? Food is still controlling our lives, and in the end, for some us, that kind of dysfunctional relationship with a Snickers bar is only going to find us waist-deep, packed with peanuts, completely unsatisfied, hating ourselves just a little bit more.

If I have to navigate through what amounts to a field scattered with land mines, I'm arming myself with more than self-loathing and shame.

I'm going in there with a sense of humor, guns blazing.

If that doesn't work, and I do wind up staring down at the bottom of an empty Pringles can, *there is always tomorrow*. I may lose today's battle, but that doesn't mean I've lost the war.

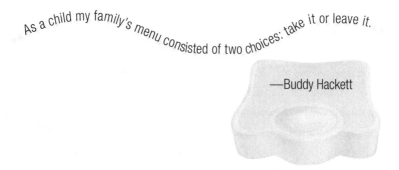

As a child my family's menu consisted of two choices: take it or leave it.

—Buddy Hackett

PMS, That Bitch
By Robyn Anderson

Tammy Wynette was right—sometimes it's *damn* hard to be a woman. A week before my period is due, I start retaining so much water that I go up two bra sizes. My breasts enter the room three minutes before the rest of me. My ankles swell so much that there's no way to tell just where they end and my calves begin. Cankles, I believe they're called. I get cranky, crabby, bitchy, and irritable (yes, we *are* blaming that on the PMS, shut up) and I don't mind telling the people (or cats) just how cranky I am, usually at full volume and with many creative uses of the word *fuck* thrown in. The day before my period starts, like clockwork, I step on the scale and I'm up 3 pounds. Three *pounds* of water, which I'm carrying around in my breasts and ankles.

And they wonder why I'm cranky.

The worst part is the cravings. Sometimes all I want in the world is a pint of Ben & Jerry's and for everyone else to go away. Other times, nothing but a huge bag of greasy chips will do. I can fight the cravings for only so long before I have to give in to some extent, or I will completely lose my mind.

You'd think that knowing that the cravings are caused by PMS would somehow help lessen them. But I can know the PMS is coming, I can give myself any number of pep talks, and I can convince myself that I don't need that nasty food, but when it comes down to it, if you get between me and Ben & Jerry's, I'll be forced to kill you. Don't get between a PMSing Fat Chick and the food she's craving; that's all I'll say.

Okay, I'll admit that I can usually talk myself into eating a substitute—low-fat frozen yogurt instead of Ben & Jerry's, baked chips instead of the full-fat stuff, you know the drill. However, when I do that, the oddest thing happens: The craving goes away when my period starts, but when the PMS comes around the next month, I crave whatever I wouldn't allow myself the month before twice as much.

PMS, she is a bitch.

I can no longer pig out the way I once did. It's not that I've turned into one of those *horrible* people who will smugly say, "Oh, I can't eat anything with grease or fat in it. It interferes when I run fifteen miles the next morning. Luckily, I don't miss that food at *all*." I still crave the stuff I used to pig out on—cake, snack foods, chips, nuts, the usual. But I've learned that the food I fantasize about very rarely lives up to the hype when I take my first bite. The ice cream is good . . . but not worth lying in bed dreaming about it. The cake isn't bad . . . but why did I spend all that time thinking about it again? I imagine it would be like fantasizing about the hunk at work—great sex in theory, but in reality he'd be all fumbling fingers, bad breath, and burrito farts.

> Tammy Wynette was right—sometimes it's *damn* hard to be a woman.

And on the occasion I find something that is as good as I remember? I can't eat as much as I used to. Not because I don't want to, but because my stomach simply won't hold that much food anymore. I don't know if my stomach literally shrunk or I just recognize the feeling of being full sooner, but I can barely get down half of what I used to eat.

It's a little annoying when I'm so looking forward to something, only to find out a few bites later that I have to put down the fork and go lie on the couch, feeling stuffed and bloated.

Stupid stomach. I suppose I could train to eat as much as I used to, but I've vowed to never cross the 300-pound mark so long as I shall live, so I guess I won't start something like that.

It's sure fun to think about, though.

I'm at an impasse. I'm at a *long* impasse. The last time I lost any significant amount of weight was about three years ago. After losing 125 pounds in less than a year, I still have about 90 pounds to lose (I'm aiming for 150, which is probably on the high side if not outside the bounds of what the height/weight chart dictates for me) and sometimes it drives me absolutely out of my mind.

> Don't get between a PMSing Fat Chick and the food she's craving, that's all I'll say.

When the first month that I failed to lose weight came and went, I was down about it, but since I'm an optimist at heart, I shrugged and figured that it was a fluke. Another month came and went, and another, and I kept shrugging on the outside, but on the inside I was absolutely obsessed with the fact that I was doing the same thing I'd been doing all along and had stopped losing weight. I refused to believe that 1,500 calories a day, coupled with 45 minutes of exercise could sustain 230 pounds.

More time went by, and I got desperate. I cut my calories down to 1,200 a day and still the scale didn't budge. Six months of not losing weight will really piss off even the most stalwart optimist. I was eating right, I was exercising, and *nothing*. I started to give up—stopped counting calories, stopped exercising quite so regularly. The scale bounced up a few pounds and then back down, and I got even angrier.

You can only sustain anger for so long; at some point you have to give it up or it'll destroy you. After a couple of years of zealous exercise for several weeks at a time followed by a step on the scale to see that it hadn't budged at all, followed by several weeks (or even months) of *Ahhh, fuck this. I'm going to eat what I want, and I'm not going to exercise again EVER*, I came to a conclusion several months ago: I can't let it be about the number on the scale or I will lose my mind.

Eating crappy food and not exercising? It makes me feel like crap, not only mentally, but also physically. Rather than letting this whole eating-right-and-exercising thing be about the number on the scale, it's become about the way I feel. I've started keeping track of the days that I eat right and exercise and in turn how I feel on those days. And big surprise—the days that I roll my ass out of bed and exercise for an hour? I feel great. The days that I eat the way I should? I don't go to bed feeling stuffed and bloated and pissed at myself.

At the time I'm writing this, it's been ninety-five days since I got back on the eating-right-and-exercising wagon. I haven't exercised every day, but I've exercised the vast majority of those days. I haven't eaten right every single day, but I've eaten right the majority of those days. I've relaxed about this thing, because it really isn't about seeing the magic number on the scale—it's about the journey.

> I came to a conclusion several months ago: I can't let it be about the number on the scale or I will lose my mind.

It's crossed my mind a million times in the past three years that maybe I'll never lose another pound. And that would suck, but I think I could learn to accept that. If I weigh 237 pounds for the rest of my life, then I do. If I don't, I don't.

But I'll feel fucking fabulous either way.

Fitness—if it came in a bottle, everybody would have a great body.
—Cher

Emotionally Hungry
By Lori Ford

I remember knowing Thanksgiving Day was coming up and that I had to make a decision about how to handle the day. Allowing myself a "free day" was treading on thin ice, like walking over peanut brittle. One free day could land me in a crack den of bottomless boxes of Ding Dongs. Before entering my father's house I took deep breaths. I can do this. Focus on the turkey breast; it's the lowest-calorie meat there is.

Have all the dry-ass turkey breast you want, I cackled to myself, knowing what I really wanted was the stuffing mounded in thick gravy.

I'd reassure myself that stuffing is completely acceptable on a free day, a real live free day; after all, I only have stuffing once a year. Why deny yourself something you won't eat again until next year?

I had gone on a trip to New York City a few months before Thanksgiving and told myself afternoon tea at the Plaza was a free meal. For weeks I fantasized about the taste of chocolate cake in my mouth, the creamy sweetness of the frosting, the soft richness of the fluffy moist cake. When the three-tiered silver tower appeared with our tea selections, there was a petit four for each of us and only one was chocolate. My face dropped. A petit four! I waited three long weeks for a petit four. My mom, aunt, and grandmother offered up the thumbnail-sized cake, which I perched on the side of my tiny plate until I ate my tiny cucumber sandwich and well-picked over scone. I popped the adorable delicacy into my mouth and passed over my $40. Some free meal.

That was my last free meal. Thanksgiving dinner at my father's was not going to consist of anything petite. It would take every fiber of my being not to eat an entire chocolate pie myself, right out of the tin.

I filled up faster than I thought possible and snuck bites of pie every time I went to refill my diet coke. They offered up leftovers for me to take home but I knew better. Much to my relief, I not only stayed out of the crack den of confections but was also only 1 pound heavier and back on my schedule.

People describe the feeling of their muscles when they lift weights. I can feel my muscles lengthening and contracting when I'm faced with some sort of office gathering. Pizza and birthday cake immediately make me feel edgy and uncomfortable. I can feel my muscles tense. Someone will always say, "Aren't you going to have some? One piece won't hurt you." But it does. Fat Lori eats the office food and Thin Lori turns it down. You can tell exactly where my head is by how I react to an office birthday. If I offer to cut the cake and just happen to land myself an extra-large share with a huge icing flower, you know I'm probably sporting large, faded drawstring pants. If I can't bother to have even a sliver, a bikini swimsuit is in my future.

Of course, there's always that scary middle ground—or rather, just scary ground—where I high and mightily turn down the cake and stop on the way home for my own bakery cake. I'll sit in the flicker of the television and try to eat the whole thing from its carton. I'll get too full and sit back for an hour or so, waiting for my stomach to produce room for more. I'll go to bed overfull and sick and have trouble falling asleep, often promising myself this will never happen again.

It wasn't until my mid-twenties that I realized I was binging. As a kid I once ate an entire bag of Doritos and promptly threw them up, involuntarily. I thought nothing of it. I don't think I recall purposely binging until I was already near 200 pounds and suffering a broken heart when my ex-fiancé moved out. Even then I think my initial objective was only to get full. There never seemed to be enough food around me to sate this need, so I'd fill up a carryout box from a Chinese buffet on the way home from school and sit in front of the television in a blur trying to get full. I'd only succeed in going from hungry to sick and waddle my way into bed crying myself to sleep. The next day I'd stop again, hoping the cashier would think I was feeding a family off my carryout box and not just me. Again that full feeling would never come, only a dull sickness. I'd sit back looking past my carryout box to the television wishing the sick feeling would pass so I could eat more. Finally, when I moved home I went on a severe diet and lost to my goal weight. It wasn't until I decided to move out on my own that binging returned to my life.

My apartment was depressing. The beige walls seemed to wash all life out of my furniture. Any color I tried to add did nothing. It was blah and didn't feel like a home. It had cockroaches and I couldn't get rid of them. I sprayed the perimeter of the apartment and all cracks every night and would still have to kill a minimum of one bug a night, often three. The apartment was immaculate and still I'd be jarred by horrors nightly. It was here that I began my favorite binge: a Pizza Hut Meat Lovers Pan Pizza and Dreamery Chocolate and Peanut Butter Ice Cream. I'd eat my pizza first, usually watching some sort of romantic-based drama like *Ally McBeal* or *Felicity*. The more tragically romantic the show the better. I'd eat the pizza until I was beyond full and then dig into the ice cream. Changing tastes from salty and buttery to sweet and chocolate helped me convince my body that it wasn't full, that it could take some more. It felt like heaven. It felt like a drug. It was numbing. It washed every pain away. Binging could only take place when I was alone. All curtains had to be drawn. A dark room with only the television on set the stage. I liked the air conditioner up high and would wrap myself in a blanket to feel small despite my ever-growing girth. It was a dark time in my life.

When I moved into my mother's treetop garage apartment, an apartment I coveted from the day they built it, the clouds lifted. But whenever work or life would stress me, I'd be at the grocery store on the way home for a pint of Dreamery and ready to dial Pizza Hut's number when I walked in the door. I'd often rent movies and make it like a party but really it was the same sad state. These binges added a bit of hysteria to the mix because I had multiple French doors that were not covered, so I could easily have been watched or caught eating all this food. Binging was a deep, dark, silent secret. The pizza box and ice cream carton were always disposed of immediately the next day. The thought of someone seeing me through my windows or my mother knocking on my door during a binge heightened my nerves and made me eat faster and even more frantically. Still, I was not cured. Chips and salsa, homemade cookies, precooked chickens, brownies, Chinese food delivery—there were lists and lists of foods I could eat massive quantities of in the sanctuary of my tiny home.

I'm spared of my own dark, secret world of binges only when I hit the zone. The zone shoots through me like a lightning bolt. It erases all need of binging. Oh, sure, I can still taste the foods that will sedate me. I imagine the binge I could have. I even hint at it during "free meals," but it's not the same. I'm in the zone. I have an objective.

Part of dieting—and realizing your food consumption is tied to something emotional rather than physical hunger—is taking stock of your life and trying to figure out why you chose to stuff your face and then your body into stretch pants rather than eat tiny portions and prance around in tiny clothes. Something larger than chocolate is responsible. I used to be certain that it was the lack of love in my life, the lack of feeling a part of a couple that left me empty and sad and turning to food to fill that void. But now I'm not so sure anymore. I've known complete fulfillment in my love life and yet I've still turned to food for comfort, to fill me. I have turned to grazing rather than binging to keep chocolate coursing through my veins. But, really, it's one in the same.

I have to turn to something besides food to fill an unknown void. I'm still searching for something to distract me.

The Power of Negative Thinking
By Monique van den Berg

I think we—and by "we" I mean Those Who Diet—should get more credit for the things we don't eat.

If I pass up a hot Krispy Kreme doughnut, I should get bonus points. If someone offers me a slice of chocolate cake and I say "no thank you," I should automatically lose half a pound. If I refrain from eating an entire gallon of Rocky Road ice cream when I'm about to have my period, I should drop a pants size automatically. This would be *fair*. This would be *a good system*.

Somehow, it doesn't work that way. I can spend an entire day virtuously saying "no" to this and "just a sliver" to that and eating Lean Cuisines and snacking on bell pepper slices and dodging every dietary land mine known to man, but if I go home and give in to one moment of weakness and eat a cookie, or cheesecake, or something, there goes the entire day down the drain!

In desperate moments, I've eaten some or all of the following:

Expired frosting
Stale chocolate bunnies
A pan of brownies straight from the oven
Cold, rather disgusting apple pie
Half a bag of chocolate chips that have turned white
Garbanzo beans

Obviously, it's my sweet tooth that does me in. And I blame the Dutch. I grew up on Dutch food, which is not actually "tasty" in the traditional sense, or any sense, especially not when my mother makes it. Vegetables with all the life boiled out of them and rabbit stew full of gristle and sauerkraut that's semi-mushy—stuff like that. But you know what part of Dutch cuisine is good? The chocolate is good.

I remember the breakfasts of my childhood—and this is probably why breakfast is still my favorite meal. We'd have rusks with chocolate sprinkles (or colored sprinkles, or vanilla-chocolate-fudge sprinkles), or waffles with tons of powdered sugar—enough to fill every little waffle square. We'd have bread with Nutella spread (and more chocolate sprinkles), or plain yogurt with so much sugar stirred into it that it became crunchy.

My mother wasn't so big on nutrition. She would feed us liverwurst-and-butter sandwiches, and she'd let me eat butter straight from the container. We drank buttermilk. Fortunately, I outgrew that particular obsession; to this day, butter turns my stomach. And *milk should not be chunky.* Pass the nonfat, please.

It's not necessarily healthy to love food this much. It's something I face up to and struggle against every single day. What I want to eat and what I am allowed to eat never match up. And it seems unfair that the small successes—the showing of restraint under trying circumstances—can be so easily undone.

They say if you only eat when you're hungry, you'll lose weight because you are "listening to your body." You know, I listen to my body. I do. And you know what? *It's always hungry.*

The number of calories I would eat in a day, if I were given the magical power to negate calories with my mind, would be staggering. I am afraid to even add it up. I am capable of eating until I feel physically ill, and then switching food genres. (I may have just sickened myself on French fries, but I'll be damned if that will stop me from having some cookies for dessert.) I feel as if I could consume thousands of calories at a sitting.

I always wished for bulimia or anorexia—one of those weight problems that results in fashionably thin malnutrition. At least it wouldn't show on the outside, at least not in the way that overeating does. But on my worst days, I'm a binge eater. On my worst days, I forget how to say no.

I stare down into the maw of my seemingly endless hunger, and I know what I'm capable of: becoming one of those bedridden fat people who need a crane to remove them from their beds. "For breakfast this morning I had six dozen eggs and a ham." Except in my case it would be six dozen doughnuts and a ham made of chocolate.

I have the fortune (and note I don't call it "good" fortune) to work in an office with a constant stream of free food. We have a freezer that's devoted to Häagen-Dazs ice cream. We have Popsicle parties. We have Mexican buffets on our pool table. (Yeah, we also have a pool table.) We have weekly birthday parties involving cake.

When food is offered, when it is right in front of you, it is damn near impossible to say no. Especially when, like me, you lack willpower. I'm very bad at saying no when food is offered to me. Especially tasty food. Especially when everyone else gets to say yes. Especially at three o'clock in the afternoon, which seems to be the worst time of the day for me, for some reason.

Which is why, if I somehow manage to say "no thank you" to an offering of food, I think my arm flab should shrink instantaneously. Victory!

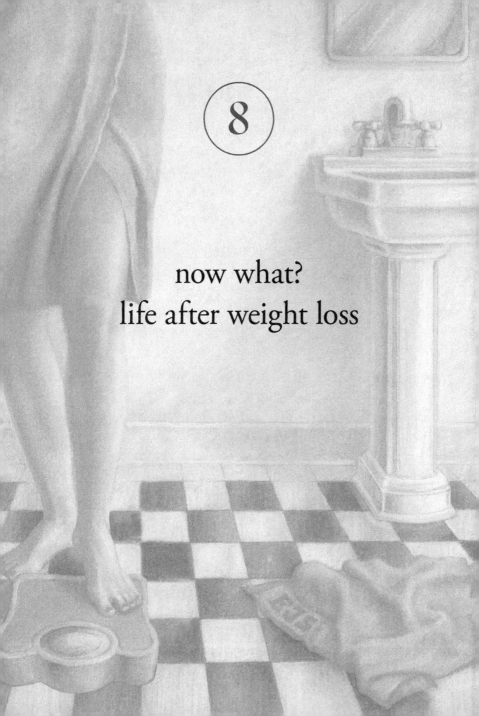

8

now what?
life after weight loss

Émigré

We're always going to be the Fat Chicks.

Yeah, that means you, too.

Even after we've Atkinsed-Weight-Watchered-starved-hypnotized-Ephedrined-Tae-Boed-Pilatesed-healthy lifestyled our safe passages to Skinnyville, some tiny font in the corner of our passports will forever read "Fat Chick."

But don't let that rub you the wrong way. It's not all bad news. After all, if the cost of living in Skinnyville gets us down or if the stretch marks betray our true identities to the natives, it'll never be too late to float on back to the shores of Fat Ass Land!

It's been more than two years since I've made the move and I've lost over 80 pounds.

So why don't I feel like a real Skinnyvillian? The reason is simple: I live the immigrant paradox. Sure, I've settled into the realm of the unfat with the intention of achieving Health and Vanity Opportunity, I have ties to Fat Ass Land that all of the promises of lard-free cookies in Skinnyville will never sever.

Immigrating to Skinnyville was something I did to better myself. Here, they do try to dress the native carrot sticks up in cute portion-controlled bags. They even go so far as to dub them "snack" packs.

In Skinnyville, there's a complex psychology that nationals must apply to the most deceptively straightforward of things. Carrot sticks aren't just carrot sticks. You're dealing with a population of people whose identities are

By Miata Rogers

wrapped up in calculating and counting everything from calories ingested to calories-burned-per-hour. It's necessary that they be spun into magical "snacks" that are so very convenient to tote around in your chic "single-serving" bag.

The Skinnyville Obsession, we'll call it, makes it easy to wax nostalgic about simpler days in the old country. Carrot cake is what it is: a delectably perfect combination of cream cheese, brown sugar, butter, and flour with a finely grated smattering of the orange root. Carrot cake doesn't need a marketing team to get the go from the Fat Ass Land public.

There's a certain kind of pride, a sense of nationalism, to be found in the Fat Ass Land immigrant community. Nothing will make you love home more than leaving it.

The immigrant paradox is always in effect and my insecurities never fail to remind me. In my mind, I'll always be the not-really-Skinnyvillian masquerading in a pair of snug, size 12 Levis, pinning my hopes for local acceptance on a pair of size 10s.

The truth is that I'm still the Fat Chick, and though I tell myself I'll never be entirely comfortable with that, I don't want to turn in my Fat Ass Land papers, either.

On good days, old relatives and friends back in Fat Ass Land try to sweet-talk me into coming back and a new Skinnyvillian coworker won't believe I've been here for "only two years!"

Despite all of this, dual citizenship is kind of nice. I can have my cake and eat it, too. That's what trips back home are for.

Comfortable in My Skin
By Julie Ridl

"You keep losing weight, and you're going to disappear!" says a colleague. She couldn't be further from the truth.

The fact is that I'm no longer invisible. I seem to be gaining more visibility every day. I'm not sure what to make of it. I'm not sure what to do about it.

Most people imagine that the feeling of losing 100 pounds must be dramatic and thrilling. It isn't. It takes quite a while to safely lose that amount of weight, and so you have plenty of time to adjust to your new, old body as the weight comes down.

In fact, losing is similar to the experience of gaining the weight in the first place. It's so gradual, you hardly notice. There is nothing uncomfortable about the process of storing fat, the outside of your pants getting smaller, and then the chair getting smaller, and then your car getting smaller.

Losing weight is no sudden relief. The changes are gradual but in reverse. Things get bigger. Eventually you adjust the seat in your car, pull the chair closer to the table, and buy smaller pants. But there is little drama. Little fanfare. Seeing people you haven't seen in a long while will bring comment, but that initial surprise is over quickly, too. And life returns to a new normal.

Except, of course, for the lack of fat prejudice. Now you get to walk through your day, meet people, joke with people on elevators, buy your groceries, buy your clothes, without having to work around or through the auto-assumptions people had about you when you were fat. Not all people, but it's certainly been proven enough times by the folks at the Rudd Institute and obesity researchers the world over that we make these assumptions.

And I know what I experienced. I know how hard I worked to climb up over my wall of fat to build credibility every day. I had the self-assurance and luxury to dismiss most biased behaviors, and working independently most of my life, I could almost always walk away from it. But for many people, prejudice against their weight is a barrier to changing jobs, gaining promotions, getting the housing they want, entering the hottest parties at the best clubs, being accepted into fraternities or sororities, even being taken seriously by their doctors. Thousands of social situations, dozens of times a day, the overweight person has to negotiate assumptions about who they are that just don't match what they know about themselves.

So now, for me, the experience of not managing all of that is a bit startling. Where I'm used to meeting people and then being immediately dismissed, overlooked, passed over, today when I meet people for the first time, there are questions. Where am I from? What am I reading? Where did I get those shoes? What a lovely handbag. I blink, and step back as if the lights are too strong. I'm not used to having this much conversation this quickly. Are you talking to me? I look around. Indeed. I often handle it awkwardly.

It's as if I've cast off a big shell, and now I feel vulnerable. I'm soft-skinned, exposed to light and rain and air. People can see me, when apparently they couldn't before. Or thought they couldn't. Or didn't want to. And so, they want to know more when they didn't before. Being left to myself, able to achieve a certain invisibility in a room, was a useful stance for an old introvert. I could observe the room. Able to look at everyone, pick up on nonverbal clues, I could sponge up the subtext of any meeting. But now, when I look at someone, they usually look back.

I can't passively observe. I'm present. People can see me.

Invisibility had its uses. Some days, I miss it. Visibility makes me conscious of my own skin and the way it fits. What pops into my head is the French idea, which roughly translated means, "To be comfortable in one's skin." My mother, who spent some of her girlhood in France, uses this expression to describe the ideal state. She uses it to describe people she admires.

Being "comfortable in your skin" is an idea that doesn't translate easily. It suggests having self-confidence, knowing yourself and knowing your capabilities, your strengths. Also knowing who you are not, and what you are not. People who are comfortable in their skin may not be, empirically speaking, beautiful at all, but they have the kind of calm confidence that makes them completely attractive. They are not easily hurt, easily thrown, easily knocked over. They are not competitive, not attention grabbing, not self-conscious.

And all that quiet confidence makes them visible in any room. You know what I mean. It explains why some people who are not classically beautiful nevertheless have great sex appeal.

It explains why so many swooned over Frank Sinatra, and why many of us faint over Willem Dafoe. It explains Drew Carey's believable love scenes. It completely explains Snoop Dog, Conan O'Brien, Rosie O'Donnell, and Isaac Mizrahi.

There are tiny, insignificant pockets of the world where attractiveness is measured in body proportions, skin tone and elasticity, age, white teeth, and big, disheveled hair. But everywhere else in the world, sexy is still measured in the qualities that actually attract mates-for-life. These are attitude, wit, confidence, trustworthiness, knowledge, wisdom.

Being comfortable in your skin means you acknowledge your past and are comfortable with your future, whether it's pretty predictable or completely open. Whether you're perfectly healthy or critically ill.

I suspect some of this kind of confidence is innate. But can't it be developed? I will tell you that merely losing weight won't give it to you. No way. That's pretty disappointing news, but better you know it now.

I can't say that I'm comfortable in my skin just yet, but I believe it's creeping up on me. I suspect I'll be there when I'm sixty or so. I'm planning to be outrageously sexy at sixty. By then I should really know what I want and don't want. By then maybe I'll stop chasing after the things that have nothing to do with who I am. I'll have cut out the distractions to focus on my real life and the things that matter most in it. Maybe I can do that by fifty. *Hmmm* . . . too much pressure.

But I've had glimpses of what it must be like. Those glimpses come in those moments when I'm thinking the least about myself and what others may think of me. They come when I'm completely engaged in someone or something else besides weight loss and fitness. When I'm excited about a new project, focused hard on learning something, engaged in someone else's story, up on my soapbox about some passion or other. It's never about the outfit or the hair. It's never about the tan or the teeth. It's never about the size. And it's never about the scale.

> A Big Mac—the communion wafer of consumption.
> —John Ralston Saul

What?

By Heather Lockwood

What am I trying to prove?

I've been asking myself that question a lot lately. Mostly when I hit the road for a long run. I'm training for a half-marathon and, in preparation, I've been spending my weekend mornings on the pavement, by myself, for up to two hours at a shot.

What am I trying to prove?

Getting ready for a run is a ritual. I rise early because I like the trail to myself. Later, it becomes crowded with the more recreational athletes. I don't know why I think I'm better than them, but I do. It is not a fair judgment, not by any means. But for some reason, I don't take people riding their bikes in jeans as seriously as I take myself.

It is 8:00 A.M. I lace up my premium sneakers. I make sure I have my water bottle pack, a radio, and a few snacks in case I need fuel midway through the run. I also wear a heart rate monitor and pedometer. I'm all about gadgets and tracking. I get a bizarre thrill from knowing my average heart rate and how many steps exactly make up ten miles.

What am I trying to prove?

Eight years ago, I would never have imagined myself a runner. I have trouble with that label now. From time to time, the subject of running will come up and my husband will say, "My wife is a runner." And for a second, I'll wonder who he is talking about. It is hard for me reconcile the woman I was eight years ago with who I am now. Sometimes, I wonder if these long runs are my penance for the past, like writing on a chalkboard: "I will never be unfit again. I will never be unfit again."

Is that what I'm trying to prove?

I knew there was a problem eight years ago. There were evenings when dinner consisted of an entire box of Rice-a-Roni. There was a serious lack of exercise. My ever-expanding pants size was entering dangerous realms. The prospect of having to shop in the plus-size section really threw me over the edge. Something had to be done.

In reaction to that, I laced up some old sneakers and headed out for a walk. Only the walk didn't seem good enough for me. It didn't seem like nearly enough effort for this sudden war on fat. I needed the big guns. I started to jog.

Of course, the jogging only lasted a minute, if that. My heart rate soared; my face turned red. This body that had been fed a steady diet of refined carbohydrates didn't know how to react. It needed guidance and training. But most of all, it needed time.

So, that is how it went. For weeks, months, and eventually years, I taught my body how to run. It started with thirty seconds at a time and grew from there. The first time I completed three miles of solid running without wanting to puke afterward, I celebrated. That was a victory because it offered hope that this recreation was actually possible. I still own my first pair of fancy running shoes because they were my first major investment in fitness: green and orange decorated Nike Airs. Those obnoxious laced-up objects actually made me want to run. They made me want to go outside and sweat and be uncomfortable and push my body to unknown levels. I'd never known such a feeling.

The running was solitary. Even though I was out there and improving, I felt self-conscious of this new hobby. I didn't dare join another person or a running group because I knew I was slow. I had no confidence in my own ability. I didn't feel like a real runner. I was just a Fat Girl who wanted to lose some weight. I remember one day specifically because my husband documented it on film. I went out for a run and, as I completed the three-mile loop, my husband popped out of the driveway and snapped my picture. When the film was developed, I didn't like what a saw: a Fat Girl in ill-fitting clothes. Her legs were marbled with red, her cheeks puffy, her brow worn from exhaustion. Instead of finding such images inspiring because of how far I'd come, I actually felt less like a runner and more like an impostor. And suddenly I was worried of what others saw when I would run past them. I could hear their comments in my head: *What is that Fat Girl trying to do? What is she trying to prove?* In retrospect, that was my first clue that I needed emotional healing, not just physical.

Running wasn't a panacea for me, either. I wish I could say it was. It didn't make me skinny. I didn't become some wonder athlete. And it was always, always hard. Even now, it is hard.

When I hear the word *runner*, I think of someone long and limber with a giant gait and an internal fire. I think of the athletes out in the rain, the athletes so dedicated that they work through pain and hunger. They glow when they sweat. They are not gasping for breath. Each stride is effortless. Each stride is easy.

I contrast that with what I think of myself running, something completely different. I am short; my gait is small. I have to concentrate on slowing my breath in an effort to control my heart rate. I do this by timing each breath with my footsteps—breathe in for two, breath out for two, in for two, out for two. My face is red. Each stride is effort. No matter how many miles I put on my shoes, it is always a challenge. It is never easy.

What am I trying to prove?

My goals are now loftier. I will soon have a half-marathon under my belt. And yet, I still don't consider myself a runner. I peck away at the mileage. I hit the trail week after week. I've spent countless miles just living inside my brain while breathing in for two, breathing out for two. During most of my runs, I think back to the Fat Girl who could barely hack it for thirty seconds. I give thanks for the ability I now have and for the training that I've done. When I pass other runners, I get a secret thrill.

But then a real runner will pass me, someone with a gait that I can't even imagine matching. The Fat Girl reappears and I feel clumsy and uncoordinated and I wonder why I'm even out there in the first place. I wonder what I'm trying to prove. Self-doubt begins to rule. And it dawns on me that no matter how many miles I put on my feet, no matter how many runs I complete, until I change my internal dialogue, I will always be the Fat Girl and will never be a runner.

Learning to run was one of the hardest things I've ever done. Training for my half-marathon has been incredibly challenging as well. But working on changing my internal dialogue is a feat I've still not managed to complete. If only it could be corrected by simply putting on miles, but it can't. I've tried that. In fact, sometimes I wonder if that is what I'm trying to prove.

Unfortunately, I don't think completing my half-marathon will make me feel any more like a runner than my first three miles did. I will continue to watch the speeds on my fellow runner's treadmills. I will continue to feel fat and slow when I am outpaced on the road. In fact, I'd wager to guess that even if I completed a full marathon, I would still have these same issues and until I resolve them in my head, no amount of mileage will fix the problem.

Perhaps this is just the lasting effect of being a Fat Girl. Once she gets in your head, she will never leave. She is always there planting self-doubt. Nothing will ever be good enough for her. Nothing will ever be enough. And as long as I listen to her, I will continue to struggle with my reconciliation between being a runner and being her.

One of these days, I will stop listening to her. And maybe my hope is that the miles will muffle her message.

The Phantom Hips
By Shauna Marsh

"What the bloody hell are you doing with your arms?"

My sister had stopped in the middle of the street and was cackling.

"What?"

"You're not that wide anymore. Your hips don't stick out that far. You don't need to hold your arms out like that!"

I caught my reflection in a shop window as I crossed the road. Sure enough, my arms were stretched out like a windmill.

"Why didn't you say something before?"

"I guess I haven't walked behind you in a while."

It's been nearly four years since I embarked on my snail's pace journey to a smaller, healthier me. As I write this, I'm 150 pounds down from my highest weight of 350. My size 30 clothes are just giant puddles of cotton gathering dust in the closet while I now manage a comfortable 14. My body looks dramatically different, but my head still struggles to believe that I take up less space.

Once I had the dreaded "morbidly obese" label slapped on me, I was convinced I was stuck with it forever. It seemed a ridiculous dream that I could ever be a remotely healthy size. I was tired, angry, resentful, and depressed. I daydreamed of miracle cures and vanishing creams, or wished for a dark van to pull up out front of my house and abduct me to a Secret Fat Camp, where a crack team of chefs, psychologists, and barking military men would whip me into shape.

But just when I'd resigned myself to a fat fate, I somehow found the energy and drive to tackle the problem. It is no exaggeration to say losing weight has changed my life, but the changes always take me by surprise, even after four years of solid effort. I'll discover I need a smaller pair of jeans or climb some stairs without bursting a lung, and I'll go *whoa* with all the bewilderment of Keanu Reeves and realize—I must have lost some serious weight, dude.

I got used to being obese. I didn't like it, but I got used to it. My whole identity was based around the blubber. My days were spent plotting my next meal, inventing lies to avoid social situations, wondering how much longer my thighs could rub together before the inner leg of my pants would dissolve completely. But by the time I'd lost 100 pounds I had to admit I was changing, inside and out. I needed to rethink my Fat Girl persona. There was a tentative new me emerging, full of energy and optimism and fiercely proud of how she'd turned her life around.

Part of me was, and still is, scared to drop the Fat Girl disguise. It's hard to let go of such a well-padded security blanket. These days if I fail at something, it's not because I'm a stupid Fat Chick; I'm just a chick now. If I don't get a job or a cute guy doesn't talk to me, I can't just blame it on the blubber. If I'm too lazy to do the laundry, it's not because of my weight—it's just because I'm just fundamentally lazy. I've lost the excuse that I constructed my entire life around, and now I'm faced with the reality of my personality.

As I write this, I'm 150 pounds down from my highest weight of 350. My size 30 clothes are just giant puddles of cotton gathering dust in the closet while I now manage a comfortable 14.

That said, I've grown to love the scariness of being smaller. I get a kick out of taking risks, not knowing if I'll succeed or fall flat on my face. It's more thrilling to try something new than to stay at home and cry into a pint of ice cream like I used to. Now I do all the little things that I used to think I didn't deserve, the things that used to make me nauseous with fear. I go to rock concerts, I run in the park, I talk to strangers in a bar, and I eat a chocolate bar in public if I feel like it. I even jumped on a plane and moved my life to the other side of the world. Losing weight has been such a grueling effort that now I am less fazed by life's other challenges. If I can drop 150 pounds, what else can I achieve? Bring it on! Life has become one big delicious bowl of opportunities, and no cream cake can compete with that taste.

> Part of me was, and still is, scared to drop the Fat Girl disguise. It's hard to let go of such a well-padded security blanket.

I am still 40 pounds away from my goal, but I am no longer obsessed by some lofty deadline. Happiness is not about my being lighter on the scale; it's about the lightness in my spirit. Happiness has come from learning to love this old body of mine right now, with all its quirks.

Now there is more to my life than fat. There is more to me than my thighs. Every day is a struggle for my mind to catch up with my smaller body, but I know I'm getting there. Some day soon I will proudly walk up the bus aisle without turning sideways to accommodate my phantom hips.

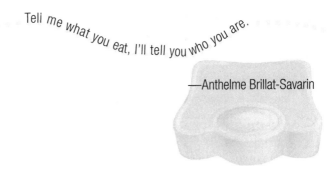

Tell me what you eat, I'll tell you who you are.

—Anthelme Brillat-Savarin

Mountain High
By Erin J. Shea

I can fit into my prom dress.

I'm compelled to let that sentence just stand on its own, resist the temptation to explain the act of being able to lift my arms and let the dress fall around my body, to zip it up without having to take a gulp of air and hold my breath for the duration.

If I have to tell you what fitting into my prom dress means—to me, to everyone around me—then instantly my ability to wear a piece of clothing is symbolic of this whole weight-loss thing. As if somehow I scaled Mount St. Fat Girl, forcefully slammed a flag into its peak, and trotted back down donning this ten-year-old cocktail dress and a smile.

But it doesn't feel as victorious as that. Wearing it now makes me feel sad, confused, *and* happy. But, maybe *for* those reasons I should tell you about wearing this dress.

Leave it to a Fat Chick to try and make a molehill out of what, to the rest of the world, is a mountain.

Buying my prom dress in England wasn't my idea, not really. Before leaving for my senior trip, my father had inferred to me that buying my prom dress while overseas would be a cool thing to do.

"You would be the only person with a dress from England," he happily said. I certainly liked that idea; I couldn't fathom wearing the sequined-splattered formal wear so popular in the United States. Besides, I could never fit into one. Surely England would have better options.

At the moment he said this to me, I still didn't have a date for the prom and the dance was a month and a half away. I had held out some hope that someone would ask me, but I knew I would have to resort to asking a friend if I hoped to go. Asking someone I had a crush on was out of the question. In actuality, it had been a year since I dared to develop anything remotely resembling a crush on a boy. Wistful, unrequited feelings for a member of the opposite sex was an exercise in abject humiliation and one I quit subjecting myself to after hearing "I'm really flattered, but I really only like you as a friend" for the umpteenth time.

Whether or not I was going to the prom was never a question. I was going to go. I had to go. Sitting at home the night of the prom would have automatically turned me into some sad little Lifetime movie character, the kind Mindy Cohn would portray with aplomb on behalf of all of the Fat Girls who had to pretend that an evening of rented movies and popcorn was actually better than a night spent awkwardly dancing to REO Speedwagon in cheap shoes. I already knew I wasn't what teenage boys' dreams were made of, but I wasn't about to solidify that knowledge for public consumption. I took matters into my own hands.

> Leave it to a Fat Chick to try and make a molehill out of what, to the rest of the world, is a mountain.

I kept track of the dance cards of my male friends like some people track football drafts, always keeping one eye on which players would be potentially called up to the NFL, with my other eye on the teams' picks. Months ahead I would single out the team *I* wanted and question him as to who *his* prospect was. If I knew that *another* team stood a better chance of signing his intended prospect, I would then let him know I was willing to step up if his prospect didn't pan out. Plus, I required no signing bonuses of any kind.

Once you told a guy you were willing to help pay for the limo *and* the after-party expenses, you looked a lot more attractive to him.

A team I had been scouting hard for myself was, by no coincidence, joining me on my trip to England. I was still unclear as to his intentions for the prom, but I knew that Mark wanted to go and somehow he didn't have a date. He and I were a small part of a huge group of people who hung out together every weekend, and nearly everyone else who comprised this group had a date.

Mark was an amiable guy: attractive, smart, and kind, the variety of teenage boy who manages to be loved by both parents and peers alike. Topping out at almost six-foot, he had sandy brown hair kept neatly in place with strategically positioned hair gel. While some guys in 1994 sported long, scraggly locks down to their shoulders, Mark's was something you were more likely to find on the head of a CEO on Wall Street. Mark's eyes were like dark stones and they shone underneath his thinly rimmed glasses—brighter still when he flashed that brilliant, wide, toothy smile he was famous for at school. Mark was more than just a great guy. He was the perfect date for a girl like me, the kind who was tired of the rejection. With Mark, there was no worrying about whether he liked me because he didn't, not in that way. As a result, within Mark's arms on the dance floor, no one questioned our coupling or why someone like him was with me in the first place.

We were friends. Nothing more, nothing less.

Midway through the trip, somewhere between a stop at Piccadilly Circus and the seventh or eighth miniature bottle of Jack Daniels my best friend Joy and I managed to purchase from the hotel vending machine and sneak past our guardians, I asked Mark to be my date. With only three shopping days left, time was ticking.

He happily accepted my offer. The next day we were scheduled to visit the ruins in Bath. It was go time.

Joy, Chelsea, and I visited a shop several blocks away from the Roman baths. In it hung a black dress made of raw silk. Delicate and light, its skirt was scalloped and it had a neckline that plunged just enough to reveal its wearer's chest without exposing her cleavage. Chelsea implored me to try it on, despite its price tag of almost $250 American dollars.

"It's a Laura Ashley," she said. "Just go for it."

As the dress fell around my body, I knew it wouldn't fasten comfortably. Without being zipped, it hung the way I would have liked—*hung* being the operative word. But as I lifted the zipper that ran up the left side of the dress, I felt the material closing in on me. The waist began to pucker and pinch. The smooth top layer of silk stretched tightly across my torso as if it would burst should I make any sudden moves. In this dress, I closely resembled one of those crocheted dolls my Aunt Hazel used to cover a spare roll of toilet paper in her bathroom—the kind that were supposed to resemble a Civil War–era Southern belle with her large skirt billowing beneath a small waist. Only in my case, I looked more like a pork sausage and the only thing underneath my waist was the fat that had been vigorously shoved downward, causing the dress to jack up two inches higher than intended.

Plus, my internal organs were fighting for space as the constrictive nature of a size 10 dress on a size 14 body forced my liver to become intimately acquainted with my kidneys, a positioning from which I'm certain they have still never recovered nor forgiven me for.

"Shea, come out and show us!"

I would have sooner jabbed rusty nails into my corneas than comply with Chelsea's request to walk out of the dressing room into the middle of this quaint English boutique so they could see for themselves what a walking, talking bratwurst looked like.

"No, you guys. I don't think this is the dress for me," I implored, hoping that I conveyed to them the right mixture of disgust and sadness with the style of the dress so that they would allow me to escape unseen.

"Well, just let *us* see," they begged. This continued for another thirty seconds until I gave up and stormed out of the dressing room, thinking that they would see the monstrosity that was me in this beautiful dress and understand my hesitancy.

I stood before them both, simultaneously screwing up both my courage and my face. They circled around me like two vultures, inspecting the dress and me in it.

"It *is* a little tight," Chelsea said. "But I bet you could fit into it by the time prom comes around!"

Joy, always the diplomat, even in the face of her friend's apparent misery, agreed and winked at me. "You can do it," she said with a smile.

I hustled back into the dressing room after their examination, knowing the decision had been made. Plus, I wasn't sure I wanted to face an entire countryside of dress fittings, sealing the fate that the remainder of my vacation would be yet another reminder of how, no matter what I did, I would never be the girl for whom the prom dresses fit perfectly.

When I got back to the States, I got to work. Exercising day and night, omitting all of my favorite foods in favor of less palate-satisfying items like water and rice cakes, I managed to make it to the middle of May without any of the nasty side effects my dieting had the potential to cause. Like fainting or death. With the help of spandex and the most unholy corseted contraption ever developed and sold in the Intimates' section of JC Penny, I wore the dress.

Mark arrived at my front door the night of the prom, corsage in hand and donning a tux. My parents took pictures and marveled at how nice we both looked together. My father even commented on our smiles, teasing us by saying that our wide, tight grins closely resembled a toothpaste ad. I glanced up at Mark and we laughed. I felt a jolt of hormones surge through my body, though I quickly squelched them to remind myself that this wasn't a date and that Mark wasn't interested in me that way, nor I him.

But as the night wore on, and I saw my classmates interact with each other romantically, I found myself more and more attracted to Mark. Every John Hughes–influenced fantasy I'd ever had crept up on me on that dimly lit dance floor and I found myself taking Mark's hand to lead him head-on into them without warning.

As we danced, I rested my head on his shoulder and felt his body tighten. Mistaking his discomfort for nervousness, I moved each of my hands to his shoulders and lifted my head to look at him. He looked down and beamed that same smile he'd flashed so many times before and quickly grabbed my hands to spin me around and do some make-shift version of the jitterbug to Whitney Houston's "I Will Always Love You." I snapped out of my fantasy, back into reality, and danced right along with him.

As we walked off the dance floor, I noticed my friends Marcia and Craig tangled up in each other's embrace and knew that no matter how much fun I was going to have that night with Mark, there would be no high school romances to look back upon and there was no way I could manufacture one for myself now.

I wasted a lot of time.

I spent my teenage years convincing myself that because I was not a candidate for the cover of *Seventeen* magazine that no boy would ever like me. I always assumed if a boy liked me at all, it was just as a friend and therefore I wasn't really attractive, at least not by the ruler used to measure good looks on women.

This wasn't true, not for all of them. It wasn't even true in the case of Wes, whom I spent the majority of my high school career pining for, assuming the reason he never wanted to date me was because of my appearance. Only when we were in college did I learn that my girth, or at least my skewed perception of it, was never a factor as much was his fear of having a relationship on the level I wanted. "I wasn't ready for something intense like that," he kindly said during a late-night conversation involving many tears and much alcohol.

Fear of rejection dominates most people's actions in any scenario and during no time is that more prevalent than in high school. But I had allowed it to so consume me that I traveled throughout my adolescence with my foot on the brake and my hands in a bag of French fries nestled in the passenger seat, all the way into adulthood. My inability to see any of the good about myself was a direct result of the considerable worth I placed on my body and its physical state.

The rest of the world wasn't measuring me by that ruler; I was.

When I recently unearthed that black silk prom dress, I'd lost 40 pounds, countless inches, and was in a panic to find a suitable cocktail dress for a formal function my husband and I were attending the coming weekend. It was only on a whim and out of desperation that I dared to try it on again, after all of these years.

I must have stood in front of that mirror for twenty minutes, looking at myself, staring back in disbelief through tears. The girl who wore this dress a decade ago was only a frightened, insecure shell of the woman who can wear it today. Being able to wear it without the aid of industrial strength control-top pantyhose doesn't bring me the kind of happiness I once thought it would. I can't turn back the clock and undo years of self-loathing and I can't make that prom dress contain a woman who hasn't been deeply affected by those years.

> My inability to see any of the good about myself was a direct result of the considerable worth I placed on my body and its physical state. The rest of the world wasn't measuring me by that ruler; I was.

But what I *can* do is let go. I can just let go. And letting go is difficult some days, especially when I catch a glimpse of my still-imperfect body at an unflattering angle. Despite having lost weight, and seeing my weight drop lower with each passing month, that girl who I was wants to be heard. She wants me to judge my self-worth on the basis of the number that appears on the scale. If I have a hope in hell of keeping the weight off and leading a life where my weight is not the predominate preoccupation of it, I cannot be defined by my weight. I *will not* be defined by my weight.

While losing weight is not easy, it's conquering my self-ingrained need for physical perfection that has been the real mountain to climb. Recognizing that there is something more triumphant waiting for me at its peak, and it's sure as hell not a set of Juicy Couture velour pants and matching hoodie in a size 4. No, it's something else.

It's just me waiting up there. That's it. Just me. And whomever she really is, inside and out, she's going to be okay no matter what size she is.

She's almost within my grasp. I get closer and closer every day.

> After all the trouble you go to, you get about as much actual "food" out of eating an artichoke as you would from licking thirty or forty postage stamps.
>
> —Miss Piggy

Still the Same
By Robyn Anderson

Of course you'll be the same person after you've lost weight as you were before.

Your bad non-food-related habits will still be there. You'll still have the same hair and eyes and that same freckle in the middle of your right palm. You'll still be the same person on the inside, with the same fears and worries, and though you'll look vastly different on the outside, you'll react to many situations in the same ways you always did.

Did you think that you'd turn into Heather Locklear, that you wouldn't leave magazines and junk mail piled up on the counter like you always did, that you'd be always calm and sweet to your family, instead of turning into Bitch Woman with no warning whatsoever like you've done your entire life? That you'd suddenly know how to dress, so that when you went out to Wal*Mart everyone would turn and stare at you and say to each other, "Who *is* that woman, that flawlessly dressed woman with that *aura* of power and confidence about her?"

You'll still be the same person whether you've lost 10 pounds or 100 or 212, because you *are* the same person. Losing weight won't change the person you are inside. It won't change that you love cats, that you prefer one cat over all others, that when it's hot and sticky outside you'd still prefer to sit on your ass and read instead of going outside to be in the sun. If you're losing weight in hopes that when you've gotten to the holy number you'll be someone else entirely, you're dreaming.

So why bother?

If someone's not making snide and bitchy comments about your fat ass or thunder thighs, they'll make bitchy comments about your nose or your frizzy hair, or the fact that every time you leave the house you're dressed like a shlump. They'll smirk about the fact that you only wear sneakers, or that you'd rather spend hundreds of dollars on books or CDs or computers instead of the finest in silk clothes and Manolo Blahniks.

Or that you had to go look up "Manolo Blahnik" to be sure you were spelling it correctly.

But here's the secret. The big bubba truth that no one ever really says: If you're losing weight for anyone but yourself, if you're losing weight because your husband or kids talk about how very fat you are, if you want to lose weight because every time you go out people stare and sneer, you're doing it for the wrong reasons.

You have to do it for you. Because your husband/kids/the people at Wal*Mart can't do it for you. You have to do it because you're tired of walking up a single flight of stairs and then gasping for air at the top. You have to do it because you can't shop for clothes at Wal*Mart, because even the largest clothes in their plus-sized section are too small for you. And because even the largest clothes in Lane Bryant are too small, and all you can wear are the largest pants from the Lane Bryant catalog, and oversized shirts from the big and tall men's catalog.

You have to do it because when you're looking for that missing cat, you have to tell your kid to get down and look under the bed, since if you got down there you might not be able to get back up without being red-faced and panting. You have to do it because every time you stuff half a box of Little Debbie Snack Cakes in your face, your kids are watching, and kids learn by example.

You have to do it because you can't walk from one end of the house to the other without needing a nap. You have to do it because if you don't, the chances are good that by the time you reach the age you consider "old," you'll either be in a wheelchair or walking with the help of a cane or walker.

You have to do it because a thousand times you've told yourself, *I'll start my diet on Monday,* and a thousand Mondays have come and gone, and you never got past breakfast.

And when you've started losing weight, when you've lost a significant amount of weight, you'll do it because there's no turning back. You'll refuse to go back to where you were, because thinking of how you lived your life when you weighed 362 pounds makes you sad. You spent your time sitting and eating and reading and watching TV, and you thought you had a pretty good life, that it didn't get much better than that.

> You'll still be the same person whether you've lost 10 pounds or 100 or 212, because you *are* the same person. . . .

So what if you couldn't fit on the rides at the carnival? It's not like you ever felt like going to the carnival anyway. It's not like you could spend hours walking around, because you'd need to stop every twenty feet to rest and catch your breath.

So what if the seats at the movie theater were too small? So what if the booths at restaurants were too small and your breasts sat on the table, in the way, and you always spilled food down the front of you because there was so much of you there that instead of falling and hitting the table, the food hit you on the way down.

So what if you and your husband didn't want to go out together, because one of you alone was noteworthy, but the two of you, at 362 and 373, respectively, caused people to turn and stare with their mouths hanging open, smirking at each other and commenting about what *that* sex life must look like.

Thinking of what life was like back then makes you sad, and you vow that come hell or high water, you'll never go back there again.

Because now you know what it's like to jog up the stairs and not be gasping for air when you get to the top. You know what it's like to be able to go out and walk 10, 14, or even 16 miles if you want. Because you've learned things about yourself—you've learned that you can fall down and get back up and keep on going. That you are stronger than you ever imagined you could be. You know that you can do it, and that you want to do it, and you feel a million times better. You sleep a thousand times better than you ever did. You look better than you did back then, and you know what? If someone wants to make fun of the way you look, or how you talk, or what you think, or those silly earrings, just smile and feel sorry for them, because they don't know. They don't know what it's like to weigh 362 pounds and then significantly less, and they're stupid, shallow people who are clueless beyond all reason, and in the end, they just don't matter.

Fuck 'em.

High-tech tomatoes. Mysterious milk. Supersquash. Are we supposed to eat this stuff? Or is it going to eat us?

—Anita Manning

A Thin Life
By Lori Ford

$\mathcal{B}$eing fat is a great security blanket. There's nothing like it. It's like I don't have to be responsible for anything. Whatever is wrong with my life is because I'm fat. I don't have to socialize, I don't have to fight for anything or believe in anything. I don't have to do anything. I can live in my own little world and block out everybody. It's safe and it's comfortable, but it's not what I want from my life. At some point I'll realize my life, the dreams and wishes I have for my life, can never come true until I give up the security blanket. Eating a piece of cake or learning to snack on carrots is not the root of the problem with me. It's so much deeper than food, so much deeper than food that ironically enough, it doesn't even involve food.

Food is the drug. Food is the means to an end.

What overeating does to me is the focus of my problem. What it means for my body, what it means for my life, what it means for my future, all balances unsteadily on what and how much I decide to eat from day to day, hour to hour. I don't know what sets off binges; I don't know what turns off "the zone" that I find so crucial to my weight loss. I don't know why what I tell myself one day doesn't work the next. It's like, one day I understand and I get the consequences of my actions. But the next day, the next hour, I could be set back for months, each day declaring, "Tomorrow, I know I can do it tomorrow, but I can't do it today. Today I must have the brownie."

I've learned there's never an end to a diet. Once the weight is gone I can never go back to the way I once ate. I suppose there's supposed to be some sort of mourning for that and perhaps if I ate normally I'd mourn that loss. But the sad fact is I don't eat "normally." I don't know what it's like to sit at a table and have a casual meal. Food elicits emotions in me that aren't healthy. I've spent so much time trying to retrain myself about food. That it's something to be enjoyed but not obsessed over. That I can eat a reasonable amount and leave the rest. That a houseful of food shouldn't make me uneasy. That I don't have to eat from the dessert menu and that eating from the dessert menu will not cure whatever ails me.

Food doesn't replace love or sex. Overeating halts my life. I know so much and have put so much into practice and yet, seemingly at a drop of a hat, I'll go back to my old ways, hiding in a pint of ice cream. I'll continue to wake up, usually months later, and get up and dust myself off and try again. I'll pick up the pieces the inner Fat Girl rampaged. I'll quell her again and fight her off again. She doesn't relent and doesn't give up and neither should I.

> Eating a piece of cake or learning to snack on carrots is not the root of the problem with me.

I have to somehow make it right with myself to be thin. It's like once I get there I pack up super-weight-loss shop and sit around twiddling my fingers. So this is what life's all about. I put myself out there, and my stomach's queasy, and everything feels so foreign. Everything feels exaggerated and not real. People are extra happy around me. Everyone pays attention to me. I squeal when I put on clothes in the morning because they fit and are so pretty and little. Suddenly everyone wants to do stuff with me. I become popular and people ask me questions. They don't look distracted when I answer them. Men linger when they look at me. It even feels uncomfortable how they want to get in my personal space, how they feel it's their right to be there.

I never had personal space issues when I was overweight. I couldn't even get a guy to have a conversation with me. Sure this experience is foreign and it's scary. Things have a way of tapering off though. The heightened excitement is gone. Everything settles into this normalcy and I still don't know who I am or where I stand. Am I still pretty today? Am I still loved today? Is my personality good enough? I start to question myself and when something bad happens I don't have weight to blame it on. This scares me. Stress returns, long monotonous workdays return, conversations lag, friends and family go back to their own lives, old problems arise, and I don't have any new answers. I feel uncomfortable and unassured and food once again beckons me to calm me, protect me, seclude me.

I have to get to a point where it's okay to be thin and still not have all the answers. That it's okay to be thin and still be lonely. Okay to be thin and still have a screwed-up life. Okay to be thin and still feel imperfect. I have to give being thin a shot as a normal part of my life, not make it a place I visit and then flee from for fear of the unknown. I need to accept myself for who I am and frolic in the joy that is size 8 for more than just a spell.

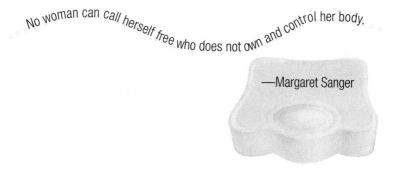

No woman can call herself free who does not own and control her body.

—Margaret Sanger

During

By Monique van den Berg

No matter how much weight I lose, or how much weight I have left to lose, one thing is certain: I am somebody's "Before" picture.

People—especially women in this "thin-is-in" society—have never struggled to find things to hate about themselves. Self-loathing: it's what's for breakfast, lunch, and dinner. And, of course, the easiest thing to hate about ourselves is our bodies.

One flip through *Cosmopolitan* magazine. One conversation with our guy friend who thinks the Olsen Twins are hot. One "You can never be too rich or too thin" bumper sticker. One look at how clothes hang on Gwyneth Paltrow. One snarky "fat ass" comment directed at someone who is 30 pounds skinnier than we are.

That's all it takes. It's easy.

Over the past few years, I have dropped probably 75 pounds and lost 10 dress sizes. But according to the BMI charts, I am still "obese." I visit weight-loss Weblogs all over the Internet and people are starting their own weight-loss journeys weighing 25 pounds less than I do. Even after having accomplished and learned so much, having achieved so much, I am still a "Before" picture.

But at the same time, I'm not. I've changed. People who "knew me when" can see it, and I can see it, too, and so can my ex-boyfriends—who I deliberately cross paths with, looking many pounds lighter and feeling, to tell you the truth, *smoking hot*.

It gets confusing, until you decide to just throw the notions of "Before" and "After" right out the window. There's no such thing.

Losing weight has taught me a few things, most importantly:

1. My dress size will never be as important as how I feel about myself.
2. If I can't have fresh-from-the-oven chocolate chip cookies every once in a while, life is not worth living.
3. There will never be a time when I don't struggle with my weight.

There will be days when I hate myself, no matter what I look like. There will be temptations and tendencies to put the weight back on. There will be fluctuations, hormonal changes, binge eating, cellulite, and most of the time, I will be the only person who cares about any of these things.

There are people who love me regardless of what size pants I put on in the morning. I could look like Chris Farley on a bad day and they would still love me. And no matter how skinny I get, I will never look like the models in *Cosmopolitan* magazine. And yet, they'll love me just the same.

> There will be days when I hate myself, no matter what I look like.

And somewhere in between those two extremes—the extremes of "fat" and "thin," which only apply in theory or in compare-and-contrast—I can be happy, and healthy, and fearless, and beautiful. I can keep trying.

Not for anyone else, or some bullshit societal standard. For myself. And just as I will never think of myself as "Before" ever, ever again, I will also never be able to think of myself as "After." I am "During." I am "Changing." I am "Learning."

I am a work in progress.

Meet the Women . . .

Erin J. Shea

Erin J. Shea is a writer and editor whose weight-loss blog "Lose the Buddha"—*www.ejshea.com/buddha.htm*—has been featured in the *New York Times*, the *Chicago Tribune*, on MSNBC.com and on the national morning show *Good Morning America*. Her work has been published in *BUST* magazine and the *Chicago Sun-Times's* Gen-X tabloid, *Red Streak*. Since launching "Lose the Buddha" Erin went from 188 to 140 pounds, changed the way she looks at food, and completed a triathlon. She lives in Chicago with her husband, Erik, and while she can now wear them if she pleases, Erin still believes pants that fall south of a woman's hips are an abomination and their creator should be shot on sight.

Monique van den Berg

Monique van den Berg lives and works in the San Francisco Bay Area, where she received her M.F.A. in poetics and writing from New College of California. Her thesis manuscript, Curves, deals with the theme of the female body. Her poems have been published in more than thirty magazines and exhibited as part of the Visual Verse project. She enjoys literature, travel, and warm chocolate chip cookies. She writes online at *http://mopie.com*.

Heather Lockwood

Heather Lockwood is a Web designer and graphic artist who lives in St. Paul, Minnesota. She shares her household with her husband and two dogs (who are treated more like children than pets). She spends her evenings writing for her Web site: *http://funnymoods.com*. When she is not writing, she can be found pursuing all things fitness-related. She is an avid road cyclist and jogger. She is also a militant health-enthusiast and proudly shops at the local co-op for all of her groceries.

Shauna Marsh

Shauna Marsh is an Australian writer currently living in Edinburgh, Scotland. She enjoys travel, pub quizzes, and watching men's tennis. Her Weblog "What's New Pussycat" (*www.shauny.org/pussycat*) has been featured in various print, TV, and radio publications, including the *Sydney Morning Herald*. She is 150 pounds lighter since starting her anonymous superhero diary, "The Amazing Adventures of Dietgirl!" at *www.dietgirl. org*. Well, not so anonymous anymore.

Lori M. Ford

Lori Ford is a self-described Very Important Accounting-Type Person, which basically means she does a lot of dull paperwork and can make an Excel spreadsheet look adorable with the right font. Her weight-loss blog, "Tales of a Bathroom Scale" (*http://dietchick.blogspot.com*) has been mentioned in the *New York Times*. A loss of 67.5 pounds has been chronicled on her blog, but at goal weight she found her weight unexplainably creeping back up. Once again she's trying to get back to goal weight and most importantly, quell the insecurities that cause her to gain weight and learn to live a life of maintenance at a healthy, beautiful weight. She lives in Wilmington, North Carolina, in an excruciatingly small but adorable apartment with her two cats.

Robyn Anderson

Born and (mostly) raised in Maine, Robyn Anderson currently lives in Madison, Alabama, with her husband Fred, teenage daughter Danielle, and a varying number of cranky cats. She spends her days in front of the computer, pretending not to notice that dust bunnies are threatening to take over the house, and her evenings rescuing small insects and rodents from the jaws of her cats. After losing 125 pounds in less than a year, Robyn hit a plateau that has lasted for quite a while—but she's pretty sure that she's going to bust through that plateau *aaany* minute now. She's had a weight-loss journal since September of 2000, which is located at *www.onefatbitchypoo.com*. She has a love-hate relationship with both her journal and her elliptical machine.

Julie Ridl

Julie blogs at *www.skinnydaily.com*, "The Skinny Daily Post." A writer and journalist, Julie G. "JuJu" Ridl lost 100 pounds. After losing the weight, she discovered the terrible truth: Maintenance takes just as much work and time. Today, "The Skinny Daily Post" is a bona fide column with a more-than-one-year life expectancy. With thousands of e-mail subscribers, and a thousand visitors a day, the Tribune Media Service's NewsCom.com sales team is busy selling it for syndication, and there's a Skinny Daily book in the works—a companion for people working to make and keep a healthy body. "The Skinny Daily Post" has been featured in papers around the world, from the *TaiPei Times* to the *New York Times*, MSNBC's Blogspotting, and iVillage's Diet and Fitness pages.